THE
CARER'S
HANDBOOK

THE
CARER'S
HANDBOOK

Essential information and support for all those in a caring role

REVISED AND UPDATED · SECOND EDITION · **2**ND

A HOW TO BOOK

ROBINSON

ROBINSON

First published in 2006 in Great Britain by How To Books Ltd

This edition published in 2017 in Great Britain by Robinson

3 5 7 9 10 8 6 4 2

A CIP catalogue record for this book is available from the British Library.

ISBN 978 1 84528 194 6

Cover design by Baseline Arts Ltd, Oxford
Typeset by Kestrel Data, Exeter, Devon

Printed and bound in Great Britain by Clays Ltd, St Ives plc

Papers used by Robinson are from well-managed forests and other responsible sources

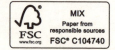

MIX
Paper from
responsible sources
FSC® C104740

Robinson
An imprint of
Little, Brown Book Group
Carmelite House
50 Victoria Embankment
London EC4Y 0DZ

An Hachette UK Company
www.hachette.co.uk

www.littlebrown.co.uk

How To Books are published by Robinson, an imprint of Little, Brown
Book Group. We welcome proposals from authors who have first-hand experience
of their subjects. Please set out the aims of your book, its target market and its
suggested contents in an email to Nikki.Read@howtobooks.co.uk

Contents

Foreword
by Judith Cameron

author of The Guardian*'s Who Cares? columns*

New parents are frequently warned that nothing they have read or been told can prepare them for the incredible demands of an infant baby. The same holds true for a person embarking on the role of carer. The big difference is that with caring, there are few guidelines, little support and vast amounts of thankless work that remain largely unacknowledged. In addition, unlike modern parenthood, becoming a carer is rarely a matter of choice.

Following a random infection of the brain that I had never previously heard of, called EL (Encephalitis Lethargica), my daughter Sophie came home from hospital eight years ago with profound brain damage. Previously a healthy and vibrant 17-year-old, Sophie returned tetraplegic, without any means of communication. She needed to be looked after 24 hours a day in much the same way as when she was first born. This time though, neither she nor I could look forward to the growing independence of childhood, adolescence and maturity.

In those early months, I felt inadequate, confused and lost. If only I could have been given a copy of *The Carer's Handbook* when Sophie came out of hospital, our lives would have been a lot easier. It would have pointed me in the right direction for a variety of amenities, as well as helped me understand the way I felt. It would have alleviated my sense of guilt at feeling depressed and angry at what had happened to my family

If asked at the time, however, I wouldn't have called myself a carer; I'm not sure I would even have stopped to think what the word meant. I already had a career and knew almost nothing about this hidden army of people that props up our health and social services. But little by little, I had to adapt and face the fact that I had become Sophie's carer. And slowly, I learned that I was not alone; that there were services and people out there who could help me, my family and her. I also discovered that like others, I did not choose to have my life turned upside down and lose my livelihood. It was not my fault that my daughter had the misfortune to fall ill.

I felt vulnerable in this parallel world of chronic illness and wished there could have been something at my disposal to help me understand my fear, sense of loss and guilt. Initially, I didn't know of people in a similar position to my own, but when I did meet other carers – of husbands, wives, children or parents – I discovered that they too felt isolated and confused. This discovery prompted me to approach *The Guardian* newspaper and write a monthly column about carers; people that society is too willing to forget.

Some time later, through *The Guardian*, I came across the original *Carer's Handbook* and was envious that I hadn't thought to write it myself. Hence, it is no surprise that when Jane Matthews asked me if I would write a foreword to this new edition, I immediately said yes. This small reference book, covering so many aspects of the work and lives of carers, is of great benefit to these unsung heroes of our times.

www.judithcameron.co.uk

Introduction

My life as a carer began without me even noticing. My uncle was diagnosed with cancer and I was the only family member with transport living close enough to help. Each Saturday the children and I drove to his home and took him to get his groceries and dry cleaning, and to the fish and chip shop for lunch.

A year or two passed and somehow the shopping trips were the least of it. As the weeks went by I became my uncle's shopper, his secretary and personal assistant, his link with the rest of the world, memory and taxi service. I ferried him to the doctors and to hospital appointments, to pay his bills, and to take his six cats to the vets. I made his phone calls, arranged for a cleaner to come in three times a week and for a home meals service. And I kept the rest of our family, geographically far-flung, in touch with his condition.

At home my two young children also wanted my time and attention. And there was the small matter of keeping my job going. The days and weeks flew by, mad, but just about manageable so long as nothing unexpected or extra cropped up. Inevitably it did. One of the children would be sick or there'd be an impossible deadline at work, or I'd get a late-night phone call from my uncle who was feeling unwell and wanted to be taken to hospital. It ought to have helped, having round-the-clock care for him in hospital. But the 50-mile round trip only made life more complicated, having to fit in time at his bedside and meetings with doctors as well as daily visits to his flat to feed the cats and tidy everything else ready for when he could come home.

1

At such times I felt like an overwound clock, the cable connecting me to all these commitments ready to snap if anyone exerted the least bit of extra pressure on it. I woke in the early hours of each morning and my brain crashed into gear, making endless lists of all the things I needed to do when day dawned.

Even things that ought to have been a pleasure, like organising the children's birthday parties, or meeting up with friends, became a chore; my heart sank every time the phone rang. Everything was just another item to add to my 'to do' list.

WHEN IGNORANCE IS NOT BLISS

Because of the way I just 'fell' into becoming my uncle's carer, it never occurred to me that I might have any choice in whether to continue. Two hundred miles away, my mother was caring for two of her aunts. Looking after family was just something you did if you were needed. At the outset my uncle made it clear that the worst thing that could happen was him not being able to continue in his ground floor flat, surrounded by his beloved cats. And none of the district nurses who came to change the bandages on his swollen legs and feet, or the hospital staff who summoned me to make arrangements each time he was ready to go home, ever suggested there might be more practical help available for us both.

There were many other things I didn't know and no one told me. I didn't know, for instance, that it was possible to get financial help towards my extra expenses. With all the extra petrol and childcare costs money was tight but no one we encountered ever suggested I might be able to claim any benefits. I didn't know about carer assessments, so when we thought that a piece of equipment or minor alteration to the flat might help my uncle with daily life he paid for it and I organised it.

I didn't know about day centres, or paid carers who might share my load. I didn't know that we were both entitled to a proper home-from-hospital plan each time he was discharged, sicker and weaker, but still determined to stay in his own place. I didn't even know who did what and therefore who I should be talking to about the myriad problems that daily life threw up.

PAST CARING

My caring role lasted five years and in that time I never once considered that I might be getting anything out of it. I felt frustration more often than I felt tenderness, and my compassion was tempered by my uncle's apparent lack of awareness of what it was costing me – and my children – to be his carers. Having lived alone most of his life he was often argumentative, opinionated and always demanding; only to the hospital and district nurses was he sweetness itself, sending me out to buy them chocolates and flowers.

Yet I can see now that we did draw close. I believe that even if he was never able to express it he found comfort in having, for the first time in a life that started in a children's home, someone on whom he could count to be there for him. I got to know my uncle and the story of his life and generation in a way I hadn't known my grandparents. And I felt quiet pride that by being his carer I was able to help him maintain a good quality of life, in a familiar setting, surrounded by the things that mattered to him, right up to the end.

Eventually, just a few weeks before he died, my uncle's cancer became too advanced for us to manage the pain at home so we moved him into a hospice. He wanted me to stay with him day and night. He seemed scared of the dark. So I asked work for more time off and spent as many hours as I could sitting by his bed. This new routine continued until, finally, I collapsed. I came home from a long shift at the hospice and sank onto the bathroom floor, unable to speak. My children called a friend who ordered me to bed and phoned the hospice to say I needed a break for a day or so. My batteries were totally flat. No longer kept alive by my energy, my uncle let go. He died late the next day.

CARING FOR CARERS

I believe that it was my friend's act of strength and kindness, putting me first, taking care of me, that saved me from breaking down completely. As carers we seem to find it almost impossible to care for ourselves the way we care for whoever it is we're looking after: friend, partner, child, parent, neighbour or uncle.

Who cares for the carer?

Try as they might, the health services, the doctors and nurses and hospitals, fail to spot that behind every person who is sick or living with a disability, or simply growing old, there is usually someone caring for them, whether or not they label themselves 'carer'. So too do the confusion of social and benefits services which make up our welfare state, too short on funds and hard-pressed to join up the dots and spot the millions of families, friends, partners, neighbours, getting on with the job, who desperately need their support.

No two carers face the same situation and yet what we need is remarkably similar: advice on what services are available and how to get hold of them. Practical help in navigating the challenges of daily life. Support in dealing with the difficult feelings which add to our load. A reminder of what choices we may still have. Even a tiny bit of recognition.

It's my aim in this guide to offer you all of those things, to make sure that as long as you go on caring you have the information and resources you need to hand. But there is something more carers need, the reassurance that they're not alone if a crisis comes: someone to 'pick them up off the bathroom floor'. That is the spirit in which this book is written, as an act of friendship and support for all of you who will recognise elements of my story in your own lives. And who need reminding that surviving life as a carer means, above all, being your own carer too.

Becoming a Carer

ARE YOU A CARER?

All her life Connie was a carer but she'd never have described herself in that way. When she nursed two husbands through terminal illness she was simply being a wife. Bringing up a daughter with a severe learning disability until she was ready to move into supported accommodation, Connie was just doing what any mother would. And all the other visits that filled her days were simply being a good neighbour.

Those whose business it is to count such things estimate that there are around six million people in the UK who could be described as carers. But nobody really knows, because of all the Connies: those who just get on with the job without ever knowing that there is a word to describe what they're doing and, therefore, that there are services to support them.

If you have a disabled child at home, if you are doing a relative's shopping or gardening, if your partner suffers periods of depression when you need to care for them, if your relative is in residential care and it's you who visits most and liaises with the staff, if your parent can't cope on their own and you're helping bring up your brothers and sisters, you are a carer.

Maybe you spend a few hours a week helping out a neighbour, a part of every weekend doing chores for a widowed parent – or you're looking after someone round-the-clock, three hundred and sixty five days of the year. Whichever it is, you are a carer.

WHY RECOGNISING YOU'RE A CARER MATTERS

It's because every carer's situation is so different that we do find it hard to recognise ourselves. It's so easy to think of other people who are having a harder time, who are having to do more. Carers who've described their lives to me always qualify any woes or complaints by assuring me they know other people who have it harder. I felt the same when I was describing looking after my uncle a moment ago. It was *only* five years. At least I was able to stay in my own home. At least I was still able to work. Carers are people who have to give up everything to look after someone else, aren't they?

Sadly, the other thing that stops us recognising ourselves is the society in which we live – one which doesn't yet recognise what being a carer means for around one in eight of the adult population. Just think:

◆ Have you ever seen a box labelled 'carer' on any form that asks for your occupation and status?

◆ At the library or bookstore have you ever spotted a section for carers similar to those for DIY or gardening or cooking or any other occupation six million people are involved in?

◆ When you chat to friends or colleagues do any of them want to know all the details of what being a carer involves for you?

◆ The last time a professional spoke to you about the person you're caring for, did they ask 'and how are you?'

The reason it matters that we are invisible to ourselves and to the world at large is because – whether you do it for 90 minutes or 90 hours – caring is one of the most important jobs there is. And like every vital job, it can be stressful, demanding, lonely and challenging. (It can be rewarding too but that's not such a 'given' as the other things on the list.) People in stressful jobs require support, yet we'll go on until we reach crisis point and only then will we reach out – when it may already be too late.

Whatever your circumstances, the moment the 'hey, I'm a carer' light goes on over your head is the moment you get the chance to start caring for yourself too.

UNDERSTANDING HOW YOU GOT HERE

Becoming a carer is a bit like crossing a road without a kerb. Normally the kerb is our signal to stop, pay attention, look around us and decide when it is safe to cross.

When there is no kerb it's hard to say where the journey begins. We are underway before we realise it, suddenly aware of cars hurtling towards us. We may glance back and see we're no longer on familiar territory, but we're most likely to keep our eyes firmly fixed on dealing with the here and now. There's no point looking ahead because there's no kerb there either to show us where this precarious journey ends.

For Graeme, there was no single moment that turned life turned upside down. Instead, he found himself simply taking on more and more for his widowed father. 'I didn't wake up one morning and think that's it. I'll be his carer. But when I met up with friends I'd realise that I didn't have much to talk about apart from looking after Dad. Apart from getting up and going to work that was all I did. There wasn't time for anything else.'

'You don't choose it. It chooses you', is how Shirley puts it. She gave up a teaching career to nurse her partner when he was paralysed from the neck down in a road accident. 'It was never a question of choice. The hospital said Gerry wouldn't walk so I just got on and fixed things at home so I could take over.'

By and large we don't choose to be carers. Like Graeme and Shirley it's something life thrusts on us. Something we do out of love for the person we're caring for, out of a sense of duty or social responsibility – or because we think no one else will. In every life things happen and we do our best to cope.

Think back. How did *you* get here? Do you feel as if you had a choice?

YOUR CHOICE TO CARE

The issue of choice is an important one. We all know that moving house is one of the most stressful experiences we can put ourselves through. And what causes that stress is similar to what makes being a carer so stressful: the sense that events are out of our control. Things that affect our lives profoundly depend entirely on the actions and choices of others. We feel stress most acutely when we believe we have no control over our own lives.

Now you're beginning to recognise that you are a carer, thinking about how you got here, and why you do what you do, may help you to take back a little of that control. When we say we have no choice we are forgetting who we are, forgetting that a sense of duty, feelings of compassion or love, a belief in the importance of neighbourliness or in families sticking together, are very much choices.

These are your priorities, the things you value above others in your life. If tomorrow you wake up and decide you can't go on then someone else will *have* to pick up the pieces, however imperfect, inconvenient or inadequate that might be. Each day you wake up and continue with the business of being a carer you are re-asserting your values, what it is that makes you, you . . . and makes the world a better place for all of us.

YOU ARE NOT ALONE

You may be feeling alone or isolated – but, ironically, you're not the only one, as the statistics show.

CARING BY NUMBERS

◆ Around six million people in the UK are carers – looking after ill, disabled or elderly partners, children, relatives, friends and neighbours.

◆ That works out at one in eight adults, doing anything from looking after someone's home or garden to nursing a loved one around the clock.

◆ With two million people becoming carers every year, by the age of 75 two in three women and one in two men will have been a carer.

◆ According to the 2001 Census, of these millions, 1.75 million care for more than 20 hours a week, of which almost one million care for over 50 hours each week.

WHY CARE? WHAT OTHER CARERS SAY

'Mum and I had a massive row and in the middle of it she shouted "why are you doing this anyway?" It stopped me in my tracks; we didn't have the kind of relationship where we spoke about serious stuff. I mumbled something about wanting to help her, helping her stay in her home, about knowing she'd do the same for me. She didn't say anything for a while but she was shaking her head. "You do it because we love each other," she said and I realised she was right. That was what it was about.' **Michelle**

'Towards the end he was lying in bed and he said "I'm so sorry you've got to look after me." I said you would do this for me wouldn't you and he said yes. So I said well I'm doing it for you.' **Taylor**

'It's sad to see her but it's not anything I can't cope with. When we got married we said for better or worse and it's turned out to be worse. That's how it is.' **David**

'I'm a great believer in family and I suppose I feel I have done my duty. I wouldn't have felt right if it was someone else doing the caring. I was able to be a stay at home parent for the children and perhaps that was an advantage in that we were all very close.' **Tony**

'It's not so bad. After all, we're all caring not because we want to or because we have to but because there are people that we love and we'd never desert them. We do it because we love them.' **Jenny**

Finding Your Way Through the Care Maze

For most things in life, there's somewhere you can go to get help and information from experts. If you are going to move house you visit an estate agent who'll guide you through the process. If you want to book a holiday, the travel agent will take the strain (and your money), sorting out all the details, the phone calls and the bureaucracy.

Caring's not like that. Instead of a single shop you're confronted with a maze of arcades offering different routes, uncertain choices, and no route map from one to another. No wonder so many carers take one look and decide to walk right on by, choosing to look after their loved one without ever coming into contact with any of the statutory agencies who might be able to help them. According to some surveys as many as two out of three carers are not known to social care services, and at least one-third aren't known to any of the health services. That's an awful lot of people 'missing in action' considering that, between them, health and social services form the gateway to a whole range of support services.

WHY SOME CARERS CHOOSE LIFE OUTSIDE THE MAZE

The most obvious reason carers don't ask for help is because they don't know they can. In a society where six million people are invisible no one thinks to tell you. You simply don't know the maze exists.

Then there's the time factor. You've already got your hands full being a carer. You haven't got time for appointments and meetings, form-filling and telephone calls. You may have put a toe in the water, contacted your doctor or social services to see if you can get any support and been put off by the reaction you got, or by someone's failure to follow up your cry for help.

Some carers fear that bringing in outside agencies will mean giving up what little control they have. You think the moment health or social services poke their heads round the door you'll be having to do someone else's bidding. You may even – heaven forbid – be found wanting, a not-good-enough carer.

And then there are those who feel that bringing in outside help is an admission of failure. Tony was like that, coping alone with the awesome task of caring not only for his severely disabled wife, but also for their daughter with Down's syndrome. He says: 'Being a male carer I was seen by everyone as being in charge, as coping, while inside I was screaming. I wasn't good at asking for help – but if I had asked I would have seen that as me failing. It was up to me to look after them.'

HOW TO AVOID A CRISIS

The thing about Tony is that, 10 years on, he says if he had his time again he'd do it differently. 'Tell people not to do what I did. As carers we have to preserve ourselves. All the time I was getting on with it alone I neglected my own needs which could have been really nasty because being a carer is so stressful.'

You may have been nodding your head a moment ago when we looked at other people's reasons for not tackling the maze. But you probably wouldn't have picked up this book at all if you were entirely happy with the way things are.

The agencies that do offer some support to carers say it's generally only when people reach crisis point that they get in touch. But just think how much harder it is to do anything when you're in crisis, you're feeling emotional, not thinking straight and you're desperate for something to change *now*. Isn't it better to try and avoid getting to crisis point at all by getting yourself as much help as you can as soon as possible?

Let's go back to that holiday and your visit to the travel agent who takes charge of things for you. The last thing they do before you write your cheque is sell you travel insurance. When your suitcase fails to arrive at your destination you wouldn't hold back on making a claim, would you?

The situation you're in now is similar. You and your relative, neighbour, partner, friend, have probably paid national insurance for years. It's not your fault you now need to claim something back, any more than it's your failure if your suitcase goes missing. It's what insurance is for, why the welfare state was invented.

One more thing to think about: would you for a moment begrudge help to someone like Tony, indeed any other carer, now you're doing the job and know what it involves? I thought not. So why deny it to yourself?

UNDERSTANDING WHO DOES WHAT

There are three main sectors that may be able to give you practical support in your caring role: the health services, social services, and voluntary (or charity) services. From here on, I shall call them the 'professionals'. That's to save you ploughing through more words than you need to, not because you're not a professional; most unpaid carers I've met do a better job than even the most committed professional who is paid to care.

Details of who does what, and who you're likely to come across, are spelt out below.

Health services

◆ **Doctor or GP.** The doctor is your first point of contact for getting general medical advice, for referring you on to specialists and involving other health services such as district nurses. Some doctors are so on the ball they run support groups for carers or offer counselling sessions within their practices. They may also make the first contact, on your behalf, with the second sector – social services – to get them involved.

Depending on your situation, you may have to deal with two doctors: your own and the doctor of the person you're caring for. If you find one more sympathetic and helpful than the other, think about switching so you're both with the same surgery, which will save you running around. But whatever arrangements you make, do make sure you tell your doctor you're a carer. It's vital that your own health doesn't get overlooked while you're caring for someone else.

◆ **District nurse.** The doctor will call in the district nurse if the person you're caring for has nursing needs which are best carried out at home, for instance having dressings changed or giving injections. The district nurse can carry out a full medical care assessment, including an incontinence assessment, and make arrangements for health care needs to be met. He or she is also a good source of advice and training in some of the medical tasks you may need or want to do yourself, such as changing a catheter bag.

◆ **Health visitor.** If you are caring for a child or young person the health visitor will assess their health needs and make arrangements for those needs to be met, check the arrangements are working, and be your regular point of contact with the doctors' practice. Health visitors may also provide health education and advice, assist with diet plans and deal with child development problems.

◆ **Community psychiatric or mental health nurse.** The community psychiatric nurse supports people with mental health problems – and those around them – by providing advice and support, and keeping an eye on how the patient is doing under any care and treatment they receive.

◆ **Hospital.** As part of their illness or disability, the person you're caring for may need hospital treatment or be referred to **medical specialists**, based at the local hospital. These are experts in the particular condition the person you care for has, for instance in the management and care of cancer patients. Be aware that the hospital will keep an entirely different set of records from the doctor's surgery and that letters of referral are unlikely to contain much more than the bare facts, so, if it's relevant, be prepared to tell the whole story again!

◆ **Other specialists.** There is also an army of health professionals who have a broader role linked not to your loved one's condition but to its symptoms or effects. They are usually based at a hospital but can sometimes be seen at surgeries or clinics in the community. They include:

speech therapist – who offers therapy for those whose conditions affect their speech, such as stroke patients
continence adviser – who gives advice and practical support on dealing with incontinence

dietician – who will advise on staying healthy through diet and on special diets for particular conditions such as diabetes or heart problems

physiotherapist – who provides treatment and advice on dealing with mobility issues

occupational therapist – who is qualified to advise on home adaptations, equipment and practical exercises to enable the person you're caring for to live as full a life as possible. They can work with you both on re-learning skills, or finding alternative ways of doing things, in order to cope with everyday tasks. Occupational therapists work in both health and social services (see next section).

There are also the **chiropodist** (feet)**, dentist** (teeth)**, optician** (sight), **orthotist** (shoes, callipers, splints, etc.) and many more, so if you think any of these services would be useful, and no one has suggested them, talk to your doctor, district nurse or to the health visitor. Some of these health professionals may be able to make home visits if the person you care for is housebound.

◆ **Hospice.** Hospices are experts in the care of people with terminal or degenerative conditions and, though most are run as charities, referrals are usually via the health service. Many hospices also run day centres and offer respite care.

◆ **Macmillan nurse.** Macmillan nurses are specialists in cancer, in the management of pain and in providing psychological support for patients and their carers. If the person you care for is suffering from cancer the doctor, district nurse or hospital may involve the Macmillan nurse whose role is also to co-ordinate care between hospital and home.

◆ **Marie Curie nurse**. Marie Curie nurses offer expert nursing care and emotional support in patient's homes and may be available for up to eight hours at a time to give carers a break. Referrals are through your district nurse or doctor.

Social services

◆ **Social worker.** Social services departments are now more usually separated into adult care departments and children's services. They are based within your local council and are where you will find social workers, who may be called case or care workers. Whatever name they go under, it is they who are responsible for two crucial assessments: the community care or needs assessment of the person you care for, and the carer assessment – a look at *your* needs. Every local authority sets its own criteria for deciding whether someone is entitled to a community care assessment and as they're allowed to take their own resources into account, there are some big gaps in provision. However, local authorities *must* by law give you a carer assessment if you ask for one.

The aim of these assessments is to produce a care plan: a blueprint for who's doing what, what services the authority will provide, and who's paying.

Your social worker may be part of a particular team within social services, serving a certain section of the community such as childcare, care of the elderly or community mental health. But wherever they fit, it is their role to give you advice on what practical help you can get and where to go for it, benefits, and to be the point of liaison with other areas of the local council's services that may need to be involved, such as day centres, home care, education services, child health. Think of them as the care 'manager' – the one responsible for bringing it all together and keeping an overview.

◆ **Home care organiser.** If the care plan makes provision for you and the person you care for to get help in the home it is usually the home care organiser who will come in and arrange this – and monitor how the arrangements are working.

◆ **Home care assistant.** Home care assistants come into the home to help look after people or those whose condition means they're unable to look after themselves properly, and to provide cover for you, the carer. For instance, they may help with getting your loved one in and out of bed, washing, dressing, going to the toilet and with household tasks such as cooking and shopping.

◆ **Other social service provision** may include support services such as night sitting and home meals delivery, and care facilities outside the home such as **day centres** and **residential homes**. You could be offered single sessions or a period of round-the-clock care so you can have some respite. Again, the social worker and care plan are the starting points for these services.

Voluntary services

◆ **Carers centres.** Like the other groups in this category, carers centres are not part of any statutory provision though many local councils support them with funding. The 800 or so local centres and associated carer support groups in the UK are among the very best sources of information and support because they understand exactly what it's like being a carer, represent carers' interests, and have masses of experience at navigating the care maze.

If you can, contact them at the same time that you contact your doctor and social services so you can get the benefits of that experience to help you. Many carer centres also offer events where you can meet other carers, and training sessions where you'll get practical help in dealing with the day to day. To find your nearest centre contact the local library, or one of the national carer support organisations whose details are listed in the resources section at the back of this guide.

◆ **Specialist support groups.** Whatever the reason the person you are caring for needs help, from a rare genetic condition to straightforward old age, there will be a support group set up by and for people going through the same experience as both of you. That means staff, volunteers or other carers who can help you get help based on their own experiences. A few of the bigger groups are listed in the resources section: many of these are sufficiently large to have local branches which your nearest library will be able to locate for you. Others, specialising in rarer conditions, may exist only online as websites, or through telephone helplines. But don't underestimate the expertise they have which will help you shortcut some of the effort that may lie ahead.

◆ **British Red Cross.** This well-known charity can loan medical equipment such as wheelchairs, and may assist with care in the home, transport needs, and first aid training. You can find your nearest centre in the phone book or by contacting the British Red Cross national headquarters given in the resources section.

◆ **Citizens Advice Bureau.** The CAB is an excellent source of free information and advice on all kinds of things, but especially in making sense of benefits and bureaucracy. If they can't help they almost always know which organisation can, and their trained volunteers will also help you complete some of those scary forms. CABs are listed in the phone book, or contact the national parent body (see resources section).

KNOWING YOUR LEGAL RIGHTS

As you pause at the entrance to the maze it's worth knowing that you do have some legal rights, though successive governments have not rushed to protect carers' interests. Carers groups have campaigned long and hard, and continue to do so, to raise carers' profiles sufficiently to persuade the government to put more effort into supporting them through codes of conduct, formal standards of practice, and through legislation.

We'll look at what the law says about issues of work and money a little further on. Right now, it's worth repeating that the one piece of legislation you should know about is the **Carers Equal Opportunities Act** which says that carers have the right to ask their local council for a carer assessment and the council's social services department *must* carry it out – and take into account carer's wishes on employment and leisure.

Unfortunately, getting an assessment does not guarantee you'll get help. The law doesn't yet insist that the council provides everything the care plan says that you need. But the sooner you ask for your assessment, the sooner you'll know where you stand on getting help.

It is also useful to be aware of the **Patient's Charter**, for both you and the person you care for. This requires the NHS to provide services to the standards agreed in the Charter and gives you the right to complain if they're not met. Among the rights it gives patients are the right to receive healthcare based on medical need, not an ability to pay, and to be able to change your doctor quickly and easily. More useful to you as a carer, but given the status of 'expectation' rather than 'right', before a patient is discharged from hospital they should be involved in a discussion about how they will be cared for when they get home, and be kept up to date with information about this at all stages.

If you are caring for a sick or disabled child then the **Children Act** spells out the duty of the local council to provide the services you need to be able to care for your child at home and to enable disabled children to live 'as normal a life as possible'. Those services include social work support, benefits advice, home help, respite care, financial support, help to have a holiday and advocacy on both you and your child's behalf.

3

The Carer Assessment

The key thing you're looking for as you enter the maze is a carer assessment. There are several routes to most destinations but research shows that the shortest cut to getting your assessment quickly is for your doctor to refer you on to social services. If that's not practical for you, contact them direct by calling or calling in on your local council. Remember, you have a legal right to this as a carer.

WHAT HAPPENS AT A CARER ASSESSMENT?

Carer assessments are carried out by one or more social workers who will usually come to the place where you are doing your caring to talk to you and the person you're caring for. You should be given adequate time to prepare and you are allowed to bring in someone to support you if you wish. The social worker's aim is to produce a 'care plan' that will set out what your needs are, how they will be met, and by whom. This may take more than one session: the social worker may need to discuss what's possible with others or get more information from other health and social care professionals. You may be asked to think about problems and solutions that have come up in your assessment.

They will want to know about your daily routine; about the condition of the person you are caring for and their longer-term outlook. They'll want to know what areas of life are difficult for you both, about the impact of caring on you and the types of support you think will improve quality of life for both of you.

Remember that you're not on trial or being judged by these visitors. It is firmly in their interests that you continue to be a carer rather than passing responsibility over to them. So there's no need to hold back from telling them exactly how it is.

The Carers Equal Opportunities Act says it is all your needs – work, learning, leisure and so on – and not just your needs as a carer that must be considered, so be sure to think ahead about those too.

If the person you care for qualifies for a community care assessment of their own, the social worker may suggest rolling the two assessments in together. Bear in mind, though, that you are entitled to a 'stand-alone' carer assessment if you prefer. Indeed, it may be essential to insist on separate sessions, for instance if the person you care for does not even accept that their situation impacts upon you.

It's a good idea to agree with the social worker when the plan will be reviewed. Your situation might change. You may need more support, specialist advice, or practical aids which you were able to manage without to begin with.

If you have doubts about your ability to continue as a carer, about aspects of care, or about the impact on your life, you should say so at the assessment. It may be that social services can offer more in the way of support than you think. Or even that ultimately you all decide that continuing to care is not the right thing for you.

PREPARING FOR THE CARER ASSESSMENT

To ensure you get the most from this process, and end up with a plan that really does help, it's important to do some preparation. You may find it useful to keep a log for about a week before the assessment takes place. Into it write every task you do during each day, problems you haven't found a satisfactory solution to, and questions you need answers to.

Another useful exercise is to work through the checklist below and jot down all the thoughts that come up. You may find it helpful to do this with someone who knows you well and whose judgement you trust. With so much to think about you're almost certain to forget something: a friend can help you stay on track.

Things to think about

❏ Do you need help with any routine day-to-day tasks: meals, medical care, getting your loved one up or going to bed, bathing, toileting, getting dressed, getting around or out, keeping them occupied, housework, garden, looking after pets, etc.?

❏ Are there any practical aids or equipment that would make a difference to your ability to care and your loved one's quality of life, such as stairlift, ramps, handrails, alarm system?

❏ What about adaptations to your home or theirs (wherever it is the caring takes place), for instance moving a bedroom or bathroom downstairs, lowering units, widening doors?

❏ Is there information you need, for example, about your loved one's condition, about what other support services such as respite care are available?

❑ Do you need help with money, for instance are you struggling to afford to be a carer, to understand the benefits system, or with managing your loved one's money for them?

❑ Do you work and want to continue to do so and, if so, what arrangements would make this possible?

❑ Do you need relief or respite care so that you can meet other commitments in your life?

❑ How are you managing (or not) to fit care around those other commitments, for instance children, a partner, other caring responsibilities?

❑ Are you getting help from anyone else: family, friends, other relatives or neighbours?

❑ How are you coping with life as a carer: is your health being affected in any way, are you getting enough sleep, do you have enough time for you?

❑ Are any areas of being a carer causing you a lot of stress?

INVOLVING THE PERSON YOU'RE CARING FOR

Along with mustering your own thoughts and keeping your own wish list, you'll need to think about where the person you care for fits into the picture.

Unless their condition prevents them from having any meaningful role in planning their own care – for instance if they're suffering from dementia – the professionals will want to talk to them too and involve them as much as possible in making decisions. At a time when their disability, illness or condition has robbed them of their independence, it's important they are not further disempowered by a feeling that they're being sidelined or treated as a child.

If you have a good, open relationship and are able to be fairly honest with each other it probably hasn't occurred to you *not* to involve them in the arrangements that are being made. You may want to work through the checklist on the previous page with them too. That way there should be no uncomfortable surprises for either of you. You may even find they're able to suggest things you haven't thought of. Perhaps they've been longing to pursue a hobby or have friends round or take baths instead of showers, but didn't like to mention it because they're sensitive to how much you are already doing.

Not all relationships are open, however. Even in the best relationships, we sometimes stop ourselves from being honest because we are scared of hurting those we care about. And then there are all the other relationships where we don't feel we can be honest at all. Life's already hard enough without having to face the consequences of admitting to the social worker in front of your father that the hardest aspect of being his carer is the way he moans incessantly about every single thing you do and say. Nor, if you're caring for someone who's struggling to accept their dependency on you, do you want to have to publicly contradict them every time they insist they can do for themselves the tasks that you're performing.

If the person you're caring for has come through the 'school of stiff upper lips' and is uncomfortable talking about anything personal, if they are struggling with being seen as needy or dependent, or don't accept or understand that they are ill, then it may be neither possible nor wise to involve them in your discussions.

What you need to do is ask that the assessment includes time for you and the social worker to talk separately. That way you're in a position to challenge any misapprehensions and ensure your needs are taken account of alongside your loved one's.

DON'T BE A MARTYR

That's about them, but what about you? If you're a carer you're almost certainly trying to be a coper – the kind of person who may not like the way things are but gets on and finds ways of dealing with them anyway. You decided a long time ago that life isn't perfect but you're usually too busy living it to stop and wonder if anything could be different.

Copers are wonderful people because they make life so much easier for the rest of us: you say you're OK so we don't need to worry about you or help you out. The social worker is trying to assess your needs and says 'how are you' and you fix a hollow smile on your face and say 'I'm fine, really.'

Expecting other people to read between the lines is usually a frustrating experience, especially if they themselves are hard-pressed and ever conscious of their department's limited budgets. You really *are* going to have to tell it like it is. That doesn't mean you're a failure. Far from it. But it does mean there's less chance of you emerging from every encounter with the professionals feeling you've been let down because no one seems to understand how tough your life is.

Don't forget health and social services need you to do this job. If you don't, they'll have to and that's going to be infinitely more complicated and gobble up an awful lot more resources than it will to support you doing the job of carer. So tell them.

PLANNING FOR A CRISIS

There's another key reason why you should exercise your legal right to a carer assessment – and that's so you and social services have an emergency plan in place. When carers are asked what worries them most, the thing that comes up most often is what will happen to the person they care for if they are suddenly unable to continue to be a carer.

If social services have never heard of you or the person you care for then it's unlikely they'll be able to put any emergency measures in place very quickly. You need the reassurance of knowing you've discussed the 'what ifs' with them and there's a plan to continue caring if you can't do it for any reason. The carer assessment is your one – and in some cases your only – chance to be identified by social services as someone performing a vital role who may, one day, need support with it.

THE CARE MAZE: WHAT OTHER CARERS SAY

'We only found out about carer's allowance by accident. It was a neighbour who asked whether we were getting it and when we talked to social services that led on to them finding a day centre for mum. And after that the council came and put a rail up outside mum's door and a handrail in the bath and they issued her with an alarm system. If only we'd known where to go and who to see we'd have got help a lot sooner.' **Linda**

'The social worker started off by saying what a great job I was doing and was there anything else I needed. It threw me because I was struggling with trying to look after dad and the twins. I'd only brought dad to live with us because I thought it would be for a short while. I was hoping we would talk about getting him into some sort of day centre at least so I only had the children to worry about during the day. But with dad there I couldn't really say anything and I assumed if he was eligible for something like that she'd have suggested it without me bringing it up.' **Lesley**

'This nurse came in because I'd said I couldn't get mum out of bed by myself and she walked straight past me and said "how are you dear, Janet says you can't get out of bed" and mum got in a huff and says "course I can, don't listen to her" and I just thought "oh mum!"' **Janet**

'I interviewed one woman who'd given up a high-powered job in London to care for her mother. The first time we met she said compared to her old job being a carer was a doddle. Six months later she was a completely different person. She was an intelligent, articulate woman who'd tried to take on the establishment and it had reduced her to a wreck. Even people who know the system as professionals, who've worked in it and then become carers themselves, say it's a battle. This constant feeling that you are not asking for much – but you are getting nothing.' **Joyce Statham, Open University researcher**

4

Working With the Professionals

The carer assessment is likely to be only one of many encounters you'll have with those working in the 'paid' caring professions. As well as the health and social care professionals we've already looked at, you may need to contact their colleagues in housing, education, employment or the benefits offices.

For you, the needs of the person you're caring for are paramount. For the professionals, no matter how experienced, how good at their job, how committed they are to their clients, you'll be one file in a huge pile on desks groaning with work.

In order to make the most of the contacts you have with these people who can support you, there are some things you need to keep in mind.

THINGS YOU NEED TO KNOW ABOUT THE PROFESSIONALS

It's not their fault. Most of them work like trojans in difficult circumstances, earn less than others doing jobs which carry a fraction of the responsibility, and never have enough hours in the day. However, this book is about you, not them, so it's as well to go into the care maze forewarned.

◆ *They're not always great at sharing information with each other*: just because you've talked to the case worker don't expect the home care assistant to know all about your situation and what's expected of them.

◆ *They will often only answer the question you ask:* before any meeting or appointment draw up your own list of the things you need to know about.

◆ *Even in their own records they usually only look at the top page*: what would you do faced with a file as fat as a brick and only 10 minutes scheduled for this appointment? Never assume when you're talking that they have the whole picture.

◆ *Unlike you, they usually don't work weekends:* some staff are on call but they probably won't be those you urgently need to contact. When they make appointments with you they'll assume you're not working and can therefore make time to meet them during their working day.

◆ *It's the person you're caring for who is their priority, not you*: you may not be comfortable putting yourself forward but there may be times when you need to remind them that there are two of you in this caring relationship. If your needs aren't also being looked after then you won't be in a position to look after anyone else.

◆ *Mistakes happen when people are stretched and stressed:* if you think they've got something wrong don't be afraid to say so. We all make mistakes and so will they from time to time. Recognising that we've done so helps us learn and do better next time.

◆ *People talk about 'the system' but it isn't one so don't expect it to behave systematically:* as Hugh Marriott points out in his excellent book *The Selfish Pig's Guide to Caring,* the fact that you'll encounter the situations above is not a conspiracy to make your life impossible. It's just chaos!

THINKING LIKE PART OF THE TEAM

Though there may be days when you feel ignored or invisible, it's vital to keep reminding yourself that far from being on the sidelines, you are at the very core of a care team. And as part of that team you are owed the same respect and support as everyone else in it, even if, unlike them, you are not being paid for the work that you do. You may encounter some professionals who do not always see it that way or who you feel don't listen properly to you or share information. They may need to be gently reminded that as your loved one's main carer you are usually in the best position to know what will help most.

If you're able, work hard at your relationships with the other members of the team. It may not be fair but it is a fact that the better you and the person you care for are known to them, and the more you project yourself as part of a partnership, the more assistance you will get. Think back to the school classroom and how quickly the teachers learned the names of the students whose hands were always up!

When you're hard pressed it may seem easier just to get on with the job by yourself. Why should you take on the extra work of chasing them when they don't return calls or follow through the things they agreed to do? Your frustration is understandable but remember that working as a team almost always gets better results because it allows you to draw on a much wider range of skills and experience. It can also act as a check when you get too close to a situation and are not always quite able to see things the way they are or could be. If they don't return your calls, don't give up but keep trying – as one social worker said, 'it's the creaky gate that gets oiled'.

TIPS ON BEING A GOOD TEAM PLAYER

◆ Keep a note of all the useful names and telephone numbers on your home and mobile phone.

◆ Make sure you know out-of-hours arrangements. Find out who you should contact in an emergency.

◆ If you are concerned about anything, don't leave it until Friday to call.

◆ Try and find out who in the 'care team' talks to whom and what arrangements there are for information to be shared.

◆ If you don't understand something, ask them to explain again.

◆ Don't allow people to rush you; you're entitled to ask for time to think things through or find out more.

◆ Take up any offers of help.

◆ Remember that while you should expect your fellow team members to share information with you, patient confidentiality may occasionally mean they can't tell you everything.

◆ And they won't always know everything – every patient is different and things do sometimes turn out in unexpected ways.

WHAT TO DO WHEN YOU HIT A BRICK WALL

You may be lucky enough to meet only complete professionals who support you and the person you care for with skills, commitment and understanding. But since we live in the real world it's more likely that every so often you'll reach a dead end or run smack into a brick wall. If you encounter confusion, delays, lack of understanding or worse, don't be afraid to bring in other professionals to help you find a way through. A carers centre, the Citizens Advice Bureau, even your own doctor, may be able to succeed where you've been making no headway. There are more suggestions for organisations to turn to in the resources section at the back of this book.

The other tool that may help you is learning to be more assertive: how to stand your ground and push – in the nicest possible way – for what you want.

Assertiveness is not about bad manners or being aggressive. It's about valuing yourself and your opinions as much as you value those of others; and about expressing your thoughts, feelings and beliefs in a straight-forward, honest and appropriate way.

A CRASH COURSE IN BEING ASSERTIVE

◆ Use 'I' messages: 'I find it hard to plan my day because I never know what time you're coming' is more effective than 'You're always late', which will put them on the defensive.

◆ Use facts rather than judgements: 'I have been waiting for you to get back to me as we agreed at our last meeting' rather than 'You seem to be forgetting or ignoring us'.

◆ Own your feelings – it's much more powerful: 'I'm angry that they made this decision without me' rather than 'They've made me angry'.

◆ Use direct words – 'no' rather than 'I don't think so', 'yes' rather than 'that would be good'.

◆ Make sure your expression matches your message and maintain eye contact. Sometimes when we're feeling awkward we smile or look away even though what we're saying is serious. This can dilute the message!

◆ Keep your voice firm but pleasant.

◆ Write down the key points you want to make and practise them in advance so you can stay focused.

◆ Keep your posture open and relaxed, which will help you speak clearly and strongly.

◆ Listen carefully to any response and let them know you've heard what they said.

◆ Don't be scared to keep repeating your point if they don't seem to be hearing you.

KEEPING RECORDS

Finally, one of the most useful pieces of equipment you can get is also the cheapest: a file and notepaper. We've already learned that you can't always count on the other members of the care team to talk to you or each other. While I hesitate to ask you to do their job on top of the two or three jobs you are already doing as a carer, my justification is that this is about saving you time, frustration and heartache.

Every time you have a conversation, find something out, make an appointment, or get a call from someone, jot it down. You should also make a note of what's been agreed, new information, names, dates and telephone numbers, as well as keeping records of tests, results, anything new or unusual affecting your loved one, and so on.

What this means is that at least one person is connecting up all the pieces of the jigsaw. It also means that if someone fails to spot something, forgets to do something they've agreed, or needs information to help make an important decision, you have the evidence they need. Finally, just in case you should ever need to go into battle with the professionals, you have a precise record of what was agreed, when and by whom.

5

Money Matters

'When my daughter, Sophie, fell ill and needed full-time care, the last thing on my mind was my career or a salary. But now, six years later, I cannot ignore how drastically her disability has affected my life and income. Although I am not poor, luxuries that I could afford easily before have become a distant memory . . . Even with a comprehensive care package in place, it is impossible to overestimate the financial implications of having a member of the family who needs full-time home care.' **Judith Cameron writing in** *The Guardian*

Judith is not alone. On top of everything else carers have to worry about, *two out of every three* worry most or all of the time about their finances. That's four million carers trying to look after a loved one while worrying about how they will make ends meet.

It was the Carers National Association (now Carers UK) that un-covered this shocking statistic in its survey *Caring on the Breadline*. The same survey showed exactly how these worries affect carers:

◆ almost one in three carers has trouble paying household bills

◆ one in five carers is cutting back on food

◆ four out of every five carers find the level of charges for services causes financial difficulties

◆ two out of three carers think worrying about money is affecting their health

◆ four out of five carers say they are worse off financially since becoming carers.

Another survey, this time by the charity New Philanthropy Capital, found the cost of raising a disabled child is three times that of bringing up a non-disabled youngster.

THE HIGH COST OF CARING

It's not hard to see why being a carer comes at such a cost. As a carer you face the double whammy of your income dropping if you give up your job or go part-time in order to care, while at the same time your expenses are rocketing. These are the hidden costs of caring. If you're at home all day, and especially if the person you care for is frail or unwell, you may need to keep your heating on during the nine months of the year when it's not warm. If you're trying to juggle caring with running your own home, with paid work, with family responsibilities, and it's nine o'clock before you're free to sit down and eat, expensive packaged food may be your only option.

Shortage of time may force you to make other choices which come at a higher cost: doing your shopping online which means paying for it to be delivered, or at the closest convenience store rather than the cheap supermarket five miles and two bus rides down the road; bringing in a cleaner because you can't even manage a lick and a promise; or, when you get two hours' rare respite, calling a taxi to take you into town because if you wait for a bus half your time is gone.

Then add to your budget the additional costs of any aids and equipment you may need to buy: clothes that are easy to get on and off, a higher bed or chair, safety guards, incontinence pads. And what about the washing bill if the person you care for needs clean sheets every day? The list is endless and, as we shall see, the help available limited, uncertain and complicated to access.

PAYING FOR SERVICES

One other thing you need to be aware of as you contemplate your finances is that you may end up with a fantastic care plan and then learn that most of the items on it are going to have to be paid for. In most cases it will be the person you care for who is expected to pay for these services rather than you. But real life is often not as neat as the professionals would like it to be so there may be an impact on you. The social worker will want to assess how much income the person you care for has before deciding whether they must make a contribution to the costs of their care. These charges will vary according to where you live because local councils set their own levels. But the law says people can't be charged more than they can reasonably afford.

Unless you're caring for a child, in which case most services should be free, it's important you talk to the person you're caring for about money before any assessments take place. One or both of you will need to have a handle on their income from pensions, investments, benefits they may already be getting as well as the extent of their savings, and other assets such as property. It's also useful to be able to show what their existing outgoings are, in other words, how much of that total income is left by the time all the other expenses are taken into account.

A word of warning based on what some carers have discovered: the person receiving the allowance has been known to regard it as an 'income top-up' for them, rather than the means of reimbursing you for all the extra expenses you're incurring on their behalf. If this happens it may be worth asking a third party such as the benefits officer, social worker or even the doctor to raise this with them. Another option is to have the money paid into a joint account, from which you can draw expenses. We'll look at managing money in the next chapter.

KNOWING WHICH BENEFITS ARE AVAILABLE

Knowing how tough it is for carers, you might expect the authorities to at least alert you to the fact that you might be able to get some financial help. Sadly, most carers tell a different story, like Mary whose daughter has severe learning difficulties and was given a place at a special school. Mary recalls: 'Because we lived a long way from the school I didn't meet the other parents until one of the teachers arranged a coffee morning and that was when one of the other mums mentioned disability living allowance. I said "excuse me, what's that?" The others said "aren't you getting it?" So of course I applied and the next time I saw my GP I told him and he looked a bit awkward and said "oh, I always assumed you were, being a professional I thought you'd know about it".'

The 'What are you entitled to?' section below outlines the main benefits you may be able to apply for. It's not comprehensive – the rules for each benefit run into entire books just by themselves. And rules about eligibility and amounts change so often, it's always best to check the current position.

Use the list as a guide only – and do consult the experts for latest information before you apply for any of the allowances. Your local Citizens Advice Bureau or welfare rights agency are good places to start, and some carers centres have benefits advisers so it's worth trying them too. You can also now get information and apply online for Carer's

Allowance, Disability Living Allowance or Attendance Allowance, via the government's Directgov website (see resources section for details). Or call the Benefits Helpline, a government service offering free, expert advice. Details of all of these services are given in the resources section at the back of this guide.

Not only will these agencies be able to tell you what you may qualify for but they can help you fill out those cumbersome forms and collect together the evidence you'll need to make each claim.

The other important aspect of claiming financial help that such agencies can help you with is how the mish-mash of allowances and benefits affect each other. You don't want to go through all the pain of applying only to find out that what the government gives with one hand it will remove with the other – something which is especially true for those carers who decide they want to continue to work.

WHAT ARE YOU ENTITLED TO?

You

Carer's Allowance
This is the main benefit for anyone looking after a relative, friend or neighbour who is ill, disabled, or otherwise unable to look after themselves. Currently, to qualify your caring duties need to occupy at least 35 hours a week and you must be over 16. Carer's Allowance is only payable if the person you're caring for is receiving the middle rate component of Disability Living Allowance or above, or they are receiving Attendance Allowance.

You don't qualify if you earn over a set amount each week or if you are studying for 21 hours or more a week. On top of that Carer's Allowance is not only taxable but any other benefits you claim may increase or decrease as a result of getting it.

Should the person you care for die, you'll continue to get Carer's Allowance for eight weeks to allow you 'time to adjust and make plans' for your future.

Recent rule changes mean if you're over 65 you're now eligible to claim but, be warned, there are rules about the way Carer's Allowance relates to pension benefits, which may mean you qualify but don't actually receive anything. This is called 'underlying entitlement' and means that you are recognised as being entitled to Carer's Allowance but unless you are receiving a reduced state pension you won't receive any money. However, you will get money in the form of a Carer's Premium if your state pension is your only income and you are receiving pension credit.

The person you care for

Incapacity Benefit

This is a benefit for people under the state pension age who have worked but are now unable to because of illness or disability. This includes those who were self-employed. Recent changes mean you may still qualify for Incapacity Benefit even if you haven't paid enough National Insurance contributions.

Disability Living Allowance

This benefit is for disabled people under the age of 65 who find it hard to care for themselves. There are different levels of payment covering both the care that is needed and mobility needs. The amount they get depends on the severity of the disability. But getting Disability Living Allowance may make the claimant eligible for other benefits too.

Attendance Allowance

This benefit is for those aged 65 and over whose disability or illness makes it difficult for them to care for themselves. It can be used to pay for help with tasks such as washing, dressing and cooking meals. However, it does not cover mobility needs.

Constant Attendance Allowance

Constant attendance allowance is a tax-free benefit which may be payable if the person you are caring for is receiving Industrial Injuries Disablement Benefit at the 100% rate or if they claim a War Disability Pension.

Both of you

There are a range of general benefits for which one or both of you may qualify. Again, as these are constantly changing do check out the current position with one of the agencies who make it their business to help carers survive above the breadline. Among those you may be eligible for are the following.

Income Support/Pension Credit

This is paid if you have no income or your total income is below the minimum level the government estimates you need to survive. It is a 'top-up'.

Working Tax Credit

Working Tax Credit was devised to leave those on lower incomes with a little more of their wages in their pocket. It can be awarded to people working 16 hours or more a week, with an additional premium if you are doing more than 30 hours a week.

Child Tax Credit

This is for those looking after a child under 16 or, if the child is still studying, under 19. You may get extra if the child is disabled.

Housing Benefit

This benefit helps those on low incomes to pay their rent.

Council Tax Benefit

If either of you is on a low income you may be eligible for help in paying Council Tax.

Social Fund

This discretionary fund is administered by Jobcentre Plus and helps with one-off expenses such as funeral costs or winter and cold weather expenses. It offers loans as well as grants, so be sure to ask for a grants application form. If you're turned down you have the right of appeal to the Independent Review Service (see resources section).

Health Benefits

People on a low income, or because of their age or the nature of their illness, may be eligible for free prescriptions, and help with dental, eye and other health care.

PREPARING FOR A BENEFITS SESSION

However much information you take with you, it's always the crucial bit that seems to be missing, so err on the side of collecting together too much information rather than too little. You don't want to have to go through this process twice. Bear in mind, too, that as most benefits are payable to the person you're caring for, rather than to you – even if it's you who's applying – you'll need to get as much information from them as you can. Useful information to take along will be:

- details and evidence of all income and savings

- details and evidence of any outgoings including mortgage/rent

- dates of birth and national insurance numbers

- doctor's note about their condition and longer-term outlook

- any previous correspondence about benefits.

Make sure you keep a record of all correspondence and telephone conversations about money and benefits because you may not always be dealing with the same person. And if you're applying for more than one benefit you may be the only one with the complete overview.

Don't be afraid to use the helplines that are given on the 'how to fill this out' leaflets which accompany the forms. Nor to take along any questions you may still have to your session with the benefits adviser.

Finally, don't forget that if your application is turned down there's almost always an appeals procedure. They have to tell you why you've been turned down and if you don't agree with their reasons, you can make an appeal. This is another good reason to keep records of everything, and, if you can, to contact the Citizens Advice Bureau or a carers centre for advice on appealing effectively.

GET A GRANT

The Social Fund isn't the only place to which you can apply for a one-off grant to help with particular expenses. Some social services departments also give financial help towards the cost of buying special equipment or making significant changes to the house where you do your caring, so be sure to ask. Indeed if the person you care for is disabled the council is obliged to help out with a disabled facilities grant to help you make alterations which will enable them to live more independently, for instance, widening doors or altering the layout of a bathroom. Councils may also make minor works grants at their own discretion, so talk to them before you lay out any cash.

The Family Fund helps families in the UK caring for a severely disabled child living at home. If offers grants that relate to the needs of the child or young person, providing they are under the age of 15, and that the equipment or services the money is for are not the responsibility of another statutory agency.

The charity sector is the other place to consider if you are struggling to afford things that will have a positive effect on the quality of life and care you can provide. A number of charities may help you get away on holiday, with the person you're caring for, or for them alone so you can get some respite.

A few of the charities set up to support people with particular conditions have special funds to assist people in hardship, as do some of the unions and professional associations the person you're caring for might once have belonged to.

Other sources to consider are the ex-forces organisations, fundraising groups such as the Masons, and local philanthropic trusts. These are the hardest to locate since some of them try not to promote themselves in case they're besieged with more applications than they can cope with.

Your local library is a good place to enquire and will almost certainly keep a copy of the *Directory of Grant Making Trusts* in the reference section.

DECIDING WHETHER TO APPLY

I'm willing to bet that as a carer and a coper the very idea of asking for money is a tough one for you – which explains why £740 million carers benefits go unclaimed each year. You certainly won't be the first one to think that if our society valued carers at all it would make sure they were financially OK without any carer ever having to ask for help.

And then there are those of you who've already tried asking for help and encountered enough suspicion and red tape to leave a seriously bad taste in your mouth. At which point your thinking goes something like, 'Well if you're going to make it so damn hard for me, if you think so little of what I do, then forget it, I'll just get on and do the job without you, same as I have been doing for the last umpteen years.'

Your anger and frustration are reasonable but before you tear the forms into tiny pieces you might want to spare a thought for other carers. I have yet to meet a carer who wouldn't go the extra mile for someone in the same boat as themselves. Every time one of us takes on the system and wins a bit of cash or recognition it shifts officialdom's understanding of a carer's life a millimetre forward. Not much, I'll agree, but somewhere down the line, we'll have all travelled far enough for change to come. And you'll have done your bit to make that happen.

Once you've decided to apply, do so as soon as you can. Benefits can't usually be backdated. And whatever else you decide, don't hold back because you're not certain whether you qualify: if you don't at least try you certainly won't get anything.

WHAT'S A CARER WORTH?

If you're still not convinced you're worth it then calculate what your many roles would be worth if someone else was paying for your time, using the exercise below. Count up how many hours a week you spend wearing each of your occupational hats and you'll get an idea of how much you, personally, are saving the state.

You might be interested to know that national carer organisations calculate that carers save the public purse in the region of £57 billion a year. That's the equivalent of the NHS budget and more than the UK's entire defence, transport, industry, agriculture or employment budgets, though strangely, no government has yet suggested setting up a special department for unpaid carers!

What does a carer cost?

Job	Approx. hourly wage	How many hours you spend	Total 'wage bill'
Care assistant	£6.25		
Nurse	£11.75		
Cleaner	£6.00		
Cook	£6.50		
Nursery assistant	£5.80		
Housekeeper	£7.50		
Book-keeper	£10.00		
PA/secretary	£11.00		
Chauffeur	£6.20		
Gardener	£7.00		
Totals			

Source: *IDS Pay Benchmark, November 2006*

More on Money

LOOKING AFTER SOMEONE ELSE'S MONEY

If you are caring for an adult who is, or becomes, physically unable to leave the house, or mentally unable to manage their own affairs, you may have to get involved in looking after their finances for them. Not surprisingly, something which our society sets so much store by can prove to be a minefield for the best-intentioned carer. Many older people were brought up believing it's rude to talk or to ask about money, which can make getting the information you need so you can help them especially tough.

Handing over responsibility for their finances to someone else may reinforce for them the fact that they are dependent on you. And if they have lived through hard times, and struggled to manage their own money carefully, seeing it in someone else's hands can make them feel especially vulnerable. While this is going on you may have other people's issues to take account of too, like Peter who felt other family members were suspicious of him taking charge of a great aunt's money for her. Says Peter: 'It was me going in there every day to clean up and water the garden and take her into town so we could pay her bills. She was confused and I'd often pay for things then she'd forget to pay me back. That was why it hurt so much when word reached me my aunt was telling other people she didn't know where her money was going. No one said anything but I felt fingers were being pointed. It was ironic, given how much it was costing me to be a carer!'

Before such situations develop, it's a good idea, if you possibly can, to get together everyone involved for a family conference to discuss managing your relative's money. The last thing you need is to have to worry about what others might be saying. Who knows, it might even be an opportunity to enlist help from them. They could share the load by taking charge of some of the book-keeping or bill paying.

Below, we'll look at a few of the areas where you may get involved in helping someone else with their money. An invaluable introduction to some of the choices and issues you face is the leaflet *Dealing with someone else's affairs*, available from Community Legal Services Direct or as a download from their website (see resources section).

BANK AND SAVINGS ACCOUNTS

The simplest way to make getting money out and paying it in easy on you both is to open a joint account, or alter an existing bank or building society account so you are both named on it. This has the added advantage that should your loved one be too unwell to get at their money, or should they die, you, as a shareholder in the account, still have access to the money for direct expenses. Meanwhile you both get to see balances and statements and so on, so you can feel reassured that everything is out in the open.

If you don't want to go that far, the person you care for can ask the bank or building society to make you an authorised user of their account by giving you what's known as a third-party mandate. Online banking is another option that is quick, convenient, and lets you see how their finances stand without having to contact anyone or request a statement. However, for many people of all ages, dealing with their finances via the hubbub of the internet is a leap of faith too far.

BENEFITS AND PENSIONS

Social security benefits and pensions must now be paid into a bank, building society, or Post Office account. But as long as the one you care for is capable of understanding what they are doing, arrangements can be made for you to have access to the money on their behalf.

If there are no property or investments involved and you simply need access to any benefits or pensions in order to pay the bills of the person you're caring for then you can apply to the Department for Work and Pensions to make you an 'appointee'. If the money is paid into a Post Office account they need to apply for you to have your own card and PIN number in order to access the money. This is covered in the leaflet on *Dealing with someone else's affairs*.

POWER OF ATTORNEY AND COURT OF PROTECTION

If the person you care for is unable to manage their affairs or needs a significant amount of help with them, you can apply for power of attorney. This is a legal document that allows them to nominate someone to make decisions on their behalf – providing they understand what they are doing when they make the power of attorney.

'Enduring power of attorney' already exists, and allows that legally-nominated person to make decisions about money and property. However, from October 2007 the Mental Capacity Act broadens the scope of how much support can be given. People will be able to make a Lasting Power of Attorney, which also includes decisions that might have to be made about health (such as whether to have an operation) and welfare (such as where to live) – as long as those decisions are made in the best interests of whoever they relate to.

The difference between ordinary and enduring power is that an ordinary power of attorney becomes invalid if the donor becomes mentally incapable, whereas an enduring power of attorney remains effective, providing the necessary steps are taken. For this reason it has to be set up while the person you care for is still capable of understanding what they are agreeing to.

A Lasting Power of Attorney remains valid even if the person who made it later becomes 'mentally incompetent'. If no such legal arrangements have been made, the new act allows the Court of Protection, from October 2007, to appoint a 'deputy'. Again, what deputies can make decisions about is set out in the Act and is firmly underpinned by the statement that all decisions must be made in the person's best interests. The Public Guardian is there to keep an eye on deputies on behalf of the Court of Protection, which may be called in if there are any disputes.

The Department for Constitutional Affairs has produced a range of easy-to-read publications about the new Act, and *Dealing with someone else's affairs* is another good starting point. See the resources section for details of where to look.

PROVIDING FOR YOUR LOVED ONE IF YOU DIE

A major worry for those caring for children or younger relatives is how to financially secure their future if you die first. You could make a will, leaving money to them, or to another relative entrusted to spend it on your loved one's behalf and for their benefit. You could create a trust fund, nominating trusted relatives or friends to provide for your loved one's needs. Or you could consider leaving money in your will to a charity which provides specialist care for your relative.

MAKING A WILL

Making a will is another area where you may feel wary to tread, but if the person you're caring for is elderly or suffering from a terminal illness it's wise to ensure their wishes are formally recorded so they have the status of law when they die. This is particularly important if you're sharing their home or jointly own property or other assets, such as a car. You need to know where you'll stand if they die.

Because of your close relationship with the person you're caring for it's probably a good idea to pay for the will to be drawn up independently by a solicitor, although if you do decide to do it yourselves you can again get the correct forms from a stationers. For a small fee a solicitor will look after the will until it is needed. But think hard about any suggestion that they should also be an executor – one of the people whose job it is to see the wishes in the will are 'executed' or carried out. If there isn't much in the way of assets you'll probably find it all goes in solicitors' fees rather than to the people or causes that your loved one intended.

LOOKING AFTER YOUR MONEY

While you're sorting out their money, you may also need to keep a very careful eye on your own. We've already looked at why being a carer comes at such high cost: it's an added source of frustration for many carers that if they're a smidgeon on the wrong side of the safety net they find themselves unable to access almost anything in the way of financial support from council or state funds, penalised for having been careful with their money.

If you fall into that category you may well be feeling anxious about how long the demands on your limited income will continue, especially if you've had to give up a job, or at least some of your hours, in order to be a carer. Your only option is to make what money you do have stretch as far as possible, and ensure managing your finances is as convenient and efficient as you can. If you're in control at least you should be able to avoid the dangers of over-spending. Take a look at the suggestions below.

MAKING YOUR MONEY WORK FOR YOU

◆ Cancel all but one credit card. It's useful to have one for ordering online or on the phone and for when you're not carrying much cash. Having just one means only one bill and you can keep better track of how much you're racking up on it.

◆ Put absolutely everything you can onto direct debit. It feels like you're giving up control but in return you know that the same amount is going out of your account every month of the year. There'll be no horrible surprises and you can budget properly knowing what you've got left for the rest of the month.

◆ Check out cheaper energy and other services bills, and any deals that can be done by using the same provider for more than one service.

◆ Wean yourself off your expensive mobile phone and back onto the landline except for emergencies.

◆ If you have a car, could you manage with a smaller engine that will use less fuel, or, when friends ask what they can do to help, suggest they give you lifts in their car?

◆ Investigate small savings that add up to more significant sums. As the carer of someone with mobility problems you may be exempt from car tax, which frees up another £2 a week.

◆ If you've had to give up work, do you have any office or practical skills you could use to earn a little extra from home?

◆ If you think your need for money may be short to medium term and you own your own home, think about remortaging to free up some cash or negotiate a temporary reduction in repayments.

◆ Ask friends for their money-saving tips, or get a book on money management from the library.

◆ Keep a record of all your spending for at least a week. Be religious about it and write down absolutely everything. It will help you spot any areas where you could make savings and any unhelpful patterns such as spending to make yourself feel better.

If you fall into debt, seek help right away. Many areas have money advice centres, or contact your nearest Citizen's Advice Bureau for help. You can get a useful leaflet on *Dealing with Debt* from Community Legal Services (see resources section).

YOUR PENSION

If you're still of working age you'll want to think about protecting your pension while you are caring. There are a number of ways of ensuring you don't end up with a lower state pension because you've been unable to work and therefore pay National Insurance. If you're entitled to Carer's Allowance you'll receive automatic National Insurance credits towards your state pension. If you don't get this benefit you may still be able to claim Home Responsibilities Protection, payable to those caring for people in receipt of certain allowances, receiving income support, and prevented from working by their caring responsibilities. However, neither credits nor protection apply if you're a married woman who's retained the right to pay the married woman's reduced rate of NI contributions.

As with all other benefits and allowances, the situation rarely stays still for long so rather than risk missing out contact your local benefits office and ask for a copy of *State Pensions for Carers and Parents*, or download one from the Directgov website. The Pensions Service helpline should also be able to send you a copy. See resources section for contact details.

MAKING ENDS MEET: WHAT OTHER CARERS SAY

'I get Carer's Allowance but they take it straight back off me. I think I'm left with £12, something like that and it's a real struggle. My son said to me the other day "Mum, I think I should get that money you get for caring for me because you're always out." So I said "Alright son, you can have it but you'll have to use it to pay for someone to come in and care for you. The government says I have to care for you for at least 35 hours a week to get this £12.35 which works out about 37.5p an hour." He said "how am I going to do that? You best keep it then."' **Jenny**

'We looked into whether mum qualified for any help around the house but because she'd got savings it looked like she'd have to pay. I did suggest she could make her savings over to me: I was worried that we'd have other big expenses as time went by and we'd need the money then. But mum didn't understand what I meant and I didn't want to push it. It might have sounded like I was doing it for me.' **Farzana**

'We used to live on my mum's pension. That was our day to day and then I got about £39 a week for being a carer and even that was taxable. We managed by downsizing. Selling our house in London and moving to a smaller place up here. The money from that's almost gone so my next thing is to downsize again.' **Janet**

7

Working Carers

For many of us, being a carer feels like a full-time job. Yet at least half of all carers are also in paid work. Juggling eels doesn't come close to the challenge of satisfying two competing sets of demands and commitments – and that's before you've begun to try and fit in the rest of your life: family, friends, hobbies . . . quiet time?

Some decide the only way to cope is to stop trying and give up the 'day job'. Others slog on, helped or hindered by their employers. Like so much to do with being a carer, there are rarely easy choices. If you do give up paid employment, will you be able to cope on the miserly carer's allowance? And how easy will it be to jump back on the employment juggernaut if the time comes when you're able to work again? But if you stay, will your career suffer because you haven't the energy to give the job your all? Will you be thought less committed if you're always having to dash off to deal with emergencies?

Before you make any decisions you need time to find out precisely what your choices are. How flexible is your employer willing to be? How much help can you get? And you need space to think about any decision's impact on you. How important is work to the way you think and feel about yourself? What are the short- and long-term costs of keeping your job or leaving it?

DECIDING WHETHER TO STAY OR TO GO

At a time when so much is out of your hands, when events seem simply to be happening to you, giving yourself the breathing space to make an informed choice is a way of helping you feel just a little more in control. Use this checklist to structure your thinking and to help you talk your options through with those you trust and who know you well.

◆ What are your options at work? How flexible is your employer? Would a few simple changes to your hours or conditions make a dramatic difference?

◆ If there really aren't enough hours in the day, would working part-time (or further reducing your hours if you're already part-time) work for you and your employer? Is job-sharing a possibility? If your current job doesn't lend itself to flexibility is there another job you could move to, with the same employer or a new one?

◆ Do you have any idea how long your role as a carer will last? If the person you're caring for is terminally ill, could you negotiate the kind of career break offered to new parents?

◆ If you stay, what will be the effects of doing two jobs on your health and well-being? Are you the kind of person who will feel more stressed because you're worrying you're not doing either job properly?

◆ Have you done the sums to see whether you really can manage on less money?

◆ How would giving up work or cutting your hours affect your pension? Does your employer's scheme allow payment 'holidays' or can you continue to make payments privately?

◆ Depending on the kind of work you're in, will your skills quickly get out of date?

◆ Finally, how important is your paid work to you? Are you someone who needs to be involved and feeling useful? To what extent is your self-esteem tied to being good at your job?

EMPLOYERS WHO CARE

Making the right choice for you will be a lot easier if you're lucky enough to work for one of the growing number of employers who recognise the importance of a healthy work–life balance; who don't expect staff to leave their personal lives with their coats at the front door; who understand that getting and retaining good staff means meeting them halfway when it comes to flexibility.

The fact that 60 per cent of us will be carers at some point in our working lives has helped drive the shift towards more family-friendly attitudes and employment law. That's an awful lot of experience and skill to lose if the world of work doesn't find ways to accommodate today's complicated lives.

Being a flexible employer might mean anything from allowing you to use the phone for personal calls, to granting unpaid leave, renegotiating hours, or allowing you to do more work from home. Ros's employer twice adjusted her hours so she could continue to work and care. She explains: 'I was working full-time so we agreed I'd start at 7 am so I could take a three-hour lunchbreak to see mum and sort out her meal and the house. Because I was going to her after work too, the days were just too long. I was only getting a few hours sleep each night so they agreed to reduce my hours to give me enough time to do the lunchtime visit without the early start. It's on a six-month renewable basis: I didn't want to make permanent changes in case I need to go back full-time.'

A number of well-known business names are leading the way and have formed an action group, Employers for Carers, to offer advice and support to other companies and to carers. Among the solutions they suggest are:

◆ '**compress**' your day: start and finish early, or start and finish late, so you have time at one end of the day to meet your caring responsibilities

◆ '**stretch**' your day by taking a two- or three-hour lunch break to be a carer before returning to work

◆ '**extend**' your working week: spread your hours over six days, giving you shorter hours each working day

◆ negotiate an allowance of **unpaid leave** so you don't have to use your entire holiday entitlement on being a carer

◆ join the growing army of **remote** workers whose employers have provided the equipment for them to do more work from home.

If you're not sure where to start, consult your employer's human resources department, a trade union or professional association, or your line manager, to see whether the company has any carer-friendly policies in place. And if not, see if they are willing to sit down and discuss your terms and conditions to enable you to continue to work while you are a carer. You could also suggest they consult Employers for Carers (see the resources section at the back of this guide).

A LITTLE HELP FROM THE LAW

Growing awareness of people's changing needs is slowly percolating through to politicians and legislators with the result that even unsympathetic employers may now find themselves bound by law to respond to your request for flexibility.

◆ The government has introduced 'Parental leave', allowing parents of children under 5 years, and disabled children up to the age of 18, an additional leave period to look after their child, though this is usually unpaid. Currently this legislation allows an extra 13 weeks (18 for a disabled child) to be taken over five years with no more than four of these to be taken in a single year. You need one continuous year's service with your employer to qualify.

◆ You also have the right to request you work flexible hours if you're caring for a child under 6, or a disabled child under 18 and claiming Disability Living Allowance. From April 2007 the right to request flexible working was extended to also include those caring for a partner, relative, or someone living at the same address. Your employer does not have to agree if there is a good business case for turning down your request; however, they do have to give it 'serious consideration'. In every case you need to have worked for your employer for 26 weeks continuously to qualify.

◆ Employees now have the right to take a 'reasonable' amount of time off work to deal with an emergency involving a dependant, if you have worked for your employer for at least one year. This is normally unpaid, although some employers have paid contingency leave schemes to cover their staff in this kind of emergency.

◆ The Carers Equal Opportunities Act says local authorities must take carer's wishes about work into account when they carry out their carer assessment: in other words, if you want to go on working the law requires them to build a care package that will allow you to do so.

Some carers choose not to say anything at all to their employer or colleagues, for fear of being thought unreliable, less committed, or too big a risk when it comes to promotion. The choice is up to you. But unless your employer really is stuck in the Dark Ages (and sadly, such firms do still exist) you may find it a relief not to have to explain or justify your behaviour every time an emergency arises – or even just when you're on a short fuse because you're tired and worried.

REMAINING EMPLOYABLE WHILE YOU TAKE A BREAK

But what if you try to negotiate a flexible package and get nowhere? Or your caring role is so onerous you feel you have no choice but to pack up the paid portion of your working week? Before you depart, do explore whether you can get a little extra cash behind you by negotiating your departure on different terms, for instance by taking voluntary redundancy or even early retirement.

If you're likely to want to return to paid work sometime – whether to your old employer or fresh fields – see if you can set up a few systems to stay in touch. Is there a staff or professional newsletter whose mailing list you could go on? Could your former colleagues let you know about any events you could attend? Or allow you to access the staff intranet or even occasional training days?

There may also be local networks in your field of work. Talk to your local library, chamber of commerce, or branch of your union or pro-fessional association. Consider whether a distance learning course could keep you up to date. And don't forget the infinite resources of the internet, which, for those lucky enough to be online, has made staying in touch a lot easier.

One issue that many carers talk about is the effect of giving up paid work on their self-esteem. At a time when your identity is already taking a hammering from a role which requires you to park many of your own needs in order to meet those of someone else, hanging on to your sense of who you are and what you're worth can be really tough. Staying in touch with the 'you' who operates successfully in the outside world of work may help keep your self-esteem intact.

RETURNING TO WORK

Should you decide you want to return to work, or circumstances change, there are local agencies who can help with everything from professional refresher courses to job hunting and job application techniques. Many carers centres also offer practical assistance and career counselling to help you on your way; while some even help fund education and training to help you return to work.

You could also consider signing up for a course at your local college, or the Open University, which allows you to study from home and at your own pace. You'll not only be bringing yourself up to date – or even launching a new career – but you'll find studying is a great boost for your self-confidence. And while you're not in work many of these courses are free.

City and Guilds has developed an online learning course especially for carers, Learning for Living, which will not only help you as a carer but could, if you choose, earn you a qualification. See the resources section for details.

If you have given up your job – even temporarily – try to remind yourself often of the skills and experience your new role demands. And don't forget that in choosing to be a carer you are exhibiting qualities such as loyalty and commitment – qualities that are on every employer's 'shopping list'. The 'advert' below may get you thinking about how many skills and qualities you do have, and you could consider using some of these words in a future job application.

ARE YOU UP TO THE CHALLENGE OF BEING A CARER?

We're looking for an exceptional person for this vital role.
As a carer, your efforts will guarantee a high quality
of life for those in most need.

◆ You'll need boundless energy, huge stamina, and an ability to work under pressure.

◆ Your role will bring you into contact with a wide range of official and voluntary agencies so you'll need excellent communication, negotiation and listening skills.

◆ You should be able to juggle half a dozen tasks at any time, all of them important, without getting flustered. That means you're able to prioritise your workload, have the ability to make decisions quickly, and can work independently, usually without supervision or regular support.

◆ Finally, you'll have bucketloads of patience and understanding, remain motivated even when you feel you're not getting any help or recognition, and be flexible about time off (we're not able to offer much)!

WORKING CARERS: WHAT OTHER CARERS SAY

'Something had to give and that something turned out to be work. One day I thought, "that's it, I'm off." I said to myself I'll have a year off, but mum got used to me being there and after a year I realised I couldn't leave her.' **Janet**

'I couldn't work because I couldn't leave my daughter but it was hard: stressful on my health and having to live on one income when we'd been used to two.' **Devinder**

'As soon as Claire started nursery I went back to work for a couple of hours and then changed to part-time when she started school. Because my job was book-keeping I was able to work at home if she was ill or it was school holidays. Mind you, they were being so flexible about Claire it meant if it was me that was ill I would struggle into work. I didn't feel I could take time out for me too.' **Mary**

8

Caring at Home

Home sweet home; coming home; there's no place like home: home is supposed to be the place we go to escape from the pressures of the world, to take a deep breath, to be ourselves.

Being a live-in carer can change the way you think about home. From being a sanctuary it is transformed into a workplace, a pressure cooker, even a prison, no matter how much you love the person you're caring for.

With around 86% of carers living with the person they care for, anything you can do to make home work better for you both, to keep it safe, to find space in it for a bit of quiet time, will be worth the effort. Let's look at how.

WHERE SHOULD YOU DO YOUR CARING?

Of that 86% living under the same roof as the person they care for, almost nine in every ten will be doing so in their own home. Of the remainder, the majority are single adults, caring for a parent in the family home. The 14% of carers who do not live with the person they're caring for are largely made up again of young adults caring for older parents, but 58% of them visit their parent or parents every day.

Geography, or your relationship to the person you care for, may have already made this decision for you. But there are situations where you do have a choice. If so, it's important to think through how each possibility will impact on your life as well as your ability to care. Take a look (below) at some of the factors you may want to take into account, whether you are new to caring, or reviewing a situation that doesn't seem to be working.

One vital consideration should be the state of your relationship with the person you are caring for before you became their carer. If it was difficult, or caused either of you grief, do not allow yourself to think that its changed status, or spending more time together, will make things easier. The changes will almost certainly simply add to the challenges, placing you under even greater strain. Try not to feel guilty if you decide to say 'no' to sharing accommodation with the person you care for: your strength in recognising your own needs will ultimately allow you to be a better carer.

Sharing accommodation

◆ They may be able to continue to keep a loved pet.

◆ They get pretty much round-the-clock supervision.

◆ Living expenses can be shared rather than running two homes.

Both in their home

◆ They are in familiar surroundings, which is reassuring at a time when other certainties may no longer be there.

◆ Neighbours and friends can still call (and may even offer to help).

◆ If anything happens to them, will you still have a home?

◆ Do you have anywhere to escape to – a room of your own – in their place?

◆ At a time of pressure on you, you may be removing yourself from your support networks.

Both in your home

◆ It may be easier for you to continue to meet your other responsibilities.

◆ Will it have a bad impact on other family members in your home?

◆ Will there be more people on hand to share the caring role and do some of your jobs too?

◆ Carers who bring their loved ones to their homes often feel more in control of events than if they move in with their loved one.

◆ Is your home big enough or can it be adapted for care?

◆ Rather like bringing work home, will you feel there is no place to escape to?

At a distance

You living in your home but caring for them in theirs

◆ There are boundaries around your caring and the rest of your life: you leave to go back to your own space.

◆ You may be spending a great deal of time and money on travel.

◆ You may be doubling your workload – and your expenses – looking after two homes, cooking, cleaning, caring for both.

◆ Because you're not there 24/7, you may be able to get more help from the professionals with looking after the person you care for.

◆ Being able to retain some of their independence may have a positive effect on their health and self-esteem.

◆ If your loved one isn't under your nose, will this make you more anxious?

Them in a residential or assisted living setting, you caring 'at a distance'

◆ Basic care needs may be being met by others, leaving you time to devote to what your loved one really wants: conversation and attention.

◆ They meet many more people and get more interest from life.

◆ They may not be getting the personal care and attention that one-to-one care allows.

◆ Unless costs are covered entirely by social services, they may be a huge drain on funds.

◆ You may spend a lot of time and money on travel.

◆ They may have expressed a strong wish 'not to go into a home', not wanting to move away from familiar people and surroundings.

◆ You get more independence.

SOURCING AIDS TO INDEPENDENCE

By the time Mary's learning disabled daughter was developed enough to walk, she'd outgrown the baby walkers aimed at helping tots stand on their own two feet. 'I decided to buy her a doll's pram instead and put a bag of cement in it so she could walk and it would support her,' Mary recalls.

Sometimes making daily life manageable is about ingenuity and experiment. Though there are literally hundreds of companies producing thousands of products to assist carers and those they care for, don't discount the possibility that the solution may be under your nose. If you can talk to others you'll almost certainly find someone somewhere has already come up with a novel way of tackling the problem facing you. As for professional help, the occupational therapist or district nurse should be able to offer lots of practical suggestions and may arrange to loan you equipment, or even help fund important adaptations to the home.

The best source of all is probably your nearest Disabled Living Centre or, if there isn't one locally, its parent body, the Disabled Living Foundation. These charities can advise on where to find second-hand equipment, put you in touch with suppliers and often allow you to look at and test your options. See the resources section at the back of this book for details of how to contact them.

The list of equipment and adaptations you might consider is inexhaustible, with new ways to tackle common problems constantly under development. The list below is intended only to give you a flavour of what's available and get you thinking about the sorts of things that might lighten the load a little for you and the one you care for.

COMMON EQUIPMENT AND ADAPTATIONS TO CONSIDER

General
long-handled catch openers for windows
pulleys for curtains
plugs with handles
entry and door ramps

community alarm system
intercom

Hallway and stairs
grab rails along walls
stairlift
stairgate
night lights

Living room
remote controls for electrical equipment and lights
electric sockets at appropriate height
mechanical chair or high-seated chair
chair tray
mechanical grabber
speaker phone

Bedroom
tray table over bed
electric or adjustable bed
sliding doors and shelves
pressure mattress
support pillow
hoist or bed pole (to help them lift themselves from bed)

Bathroom and loo
raised toilet seat
handrails
tap levers
bath or shower seat
walk-in bath

non-slip mats
long-handled brushes
liquid soap and shampoo dispensers

Dressing
long-handled shoe horn
dressing stick
simple fastenings such as Velcro

Eating
two-handled cup
plate guard
angled cutlery
swivel seat
bibs for everyone!

While you're thinking about aids, bear in mind there's no reason the sitting room has to be where it's always been if converting it to a bedsit for your loved one would give them more independence and you a bit more space. Carers have turned laundry rooms into downstairs bathrooms, lounges into bedrooms, ground floors into first floors – whatever works for them. Even the smallest homes can be made a little more flexible with the introduction of a room divider.

GETTING ORGANISED

In today's fast-forward society, most of us feel as if we're jugglers, trying to keep all the balls in the air without dropping anything important. The following tips come from other carers who've found them useful for keeping on top of most things, most of the time.

TIPS

◆ Create a bulletin board just for those things to do with caring: important telephone numbers, appointment cards, dietary details, whatever you and others need to be able to put your hands on instantly.

◆ Keep an extra set of those things that it would be disastrous to lose: keys, glasses, photocopies of important documents such as birth and marriage certificates, national insurance numbers, alarm codes, etc.

◆ Keep everything to do with the person you're caring for in a single accessible place such as an accordion file, for instance details of medicines, treatments, their home, bills, finances, will and so on.

◆ Get a mobile phone so that you can go out but be reached in an emergency; and an answerphone at home so you can choose when to take calls and when to screen them.

◆ Get a large wall calendar so neither of you miss any important appointments or visits – then get in the habit of consulting it every day.

◆ If their health is fragile, keep an overnight bag for each of you packed with essentials such as toothbrush, toiletries, nightwear and underwear.

STAYING SAFE

We're always being told more accidents happen in the home than anywhere else – and we're always being told it because it's true. Of course you're already doing your best to keep you both safe but the busier our lives are, the more likely we are to overlook obvious things. As a carer with so much on your plate, you're more vulnerable.

Staying aware of safety means remembering some basic rules.

◆ Don't leave things lying on the floor, hallways or stairs. Invest in a big straw basket and sling in everything you need to put away but don't have time for right now.

◆ If you or your loved one have to get up at night, install a night light or put reflective tape on sharp corners and stair edges.

◆ A baby monitor is a simple way of staying aware of what else is going on in the house when you're tied up.

◆ Install smoke alarms and change the batteries every New Year's Day, without fail.

◆ You may also want to invest in fire extinguishers and teach everyone in the house how to use them.

◆ Remove the lock on the bathroom door and hang an 'occupied' sign on it instead.

◆ Get an alarm system installed, so that in an emergency you or your loved one can notify someone immediately that you need help. Most councils now have a community alarm system, linked to a team of wardens trained in emergency response.

◆ Whenever you find yourself rushing around the house, in the street, or behind the wheel of a car, actively tell yourself to 'slow down'. Rushing about really won't get things done more quickly (if you don't believe me, think how many times the guy who tailgated you then screeched past is still fuming at the traffic lights when you catch up).

CREATING A GOOD ENVIRONMENT FOR YOU BOTH

We started this section by thinking about what home means to us. More than ever for you as a carer it's important to preserve as much of that as you can. If you are living with the person you care for you need to think about what boundaries you can put in place to help you switch off sometimes: having one room or a space in a room that is yours alone, for instance, filled with the things that make you feel good and at peace. It could be a bedroom, an attic conversion, even the garden shed, so long as going in and closing the door means you are temporarily off duty.

If your home's simply too small for that to be an option, think about how you can create mental boundaries. Your home is now, after all, your workplace too. For most of us the end of the working day involves at least a short journey home, which is a useful way of closing the bracket on the day. Could you take a turn round the block or the garden when the person you're caring for goes to bed? Or get into the habit of treating every bath you have or every meal you cook as time for you, surrounded with music you enjoy and good smells?

As your workplace, and an environment in which you are both spending a lot of time, you want the home to be not only practical but a really pleasant place to be. Think about the little touches that can help make it a place of peace and interest and put them on your Christmas or birthday list:

◆ wind chimes in a doorway or patio

◆ house plants and, in the garden, perennials for year-round colour

◆ a bird feeder outside the window or low-maintenance pet such as a goldfish

◆ plenty of music – most libraries now loan a wide range of artists and styles

◆ heated packs or hot water bottles to comfort you both

◆ a teasmade – you won't always find the time to stop, but the machine will remember for you that it's time for a 10-minute break!

◆ scented candles to perfume the air.

9

Healthy Minds and Healthy Bodies

For too many carers, looking after someone has the same effect on their health as piling weights on one side of a scale. The more you put into one side, the less there is available on your side. More than half of the carers questioned in a survey for the Princess Royal Trust for Carers said their own health was not good, complaining of everything from stress (38% of carers) to back injuries (20%) to depression (28%).

Unlike being in paid work, there's usually no provision for having time off sick – so most carers don't, no matter how ill they are.

Your own health is vital. Vital in order that you can carry on, vital to your own quality of life while you're a carer, and vital so that you don't end up needing care yourself. However hard-pressed you are, you must make looking after yourself an equal priority with caring for the one you're looking after.

PLANNING A HEALTHY DIET

A good and balanced diet is important for you both, but a challenge to provide if there already aren't enough hours in the day. Rather than planning big meals two or three times a day you might find it easier to have snack stops: sandwiches, fruit, cheese and biscuits, milk shakes, soup, cereals. It's also a way of breaking up the hours if time weighs heavily on the hands of the person you care for. You can get advice on planning a healthy diet from the dietician at the local hospital or the health visitor.

Many areas of the UK do still run Meals on Wheels services: social services will be able to tell you who to contact. Or you can buy frozen pre-prepared meals from a number of private companies operating a home delivery service. They're not much more expensive than Meals on Wheels and, because the companies provide a reasonably extensive menu, the person you're caring for gets more choice about what they want to eat. Again, social services can usually give you details of the operators in your area.

Supermarkets are increasingly another source of ready meals but unless you've got lots of time for the small print you may find it harder to get a properly balanced diet. Since your own health is vital to you being able to continue to care, think about taking dietary supplements, for instance a multivitamin pill and mineral supplement. Some of these are available in energy or dietary drinks: expensive again but a quick and pleasant way of keeping your system topped up with essentials.

If you really can't face cooking at the end of the day then a couple of pieces of fruit and a sandwich will do you more good than phoning for a takeout. And food is an area where you could consider taking up any offers of help your friends, neighbours or relatives make. It's no trouble for most people to cook one or two extra portions of the meal they're preparing and save them for you.

STAYING OR GETTING FIT

You may never have been a great fan of exercise, but even if you think that pilates is a rather unpleasant medical condition, now you're a carer the way to look at exercise is as 'time out'. And don't be fooled into convincing yourself all that running around, up and down stairs, between home and work, to the shops and appointments, is keeping you fit: activity under stress is almost worse than no activity at all. Your body is wound like a spring and liable to snap altogether.

The best thing about 'formal' exercise is that it has a positive effect on your mind as well as your body. Methods such as yoga or t'ai chi actually train your mind to be still for a while, at the same time as your body is being gently stretched. Even a hectic game of squash, badminton or other competitive sport has a relaxing effect on both body and mind because it requires concentration. And thinking about the game temporarily squeezes out the million other things that concern you as a carer. Whether you choose jogging, brisk walking, swimming, a keep-fit class, or a trip to the gym, the most helpful form of exercise will take you out of the home and among other people.

If the only way you can get out is by taking the person you care for with you – and their health allows it – then do so. The time out will still be good for your health. But if you really are housebound then there are exercise videos you can follow from home, guiding you through sessions in keep fit or yoga. Most libraries keep a stock. Alternatively, you could draw the curtains, put on your favourite upbeat music and throw yourself around for 15 minutes. Dancing is great exercise and you will feel more alive by the time you're done.

If physical activity is out of the question for the person you're caring for, consult their doctor or the occupational therapist. Immobility only leads to more health problems and there are exercises that can be performed in a chair, from rotating joints – wrists, ankles and neck – to stretching. This can also help break up the day for those whose age or disability keeps them pretty much confined to home.

OBSERVING BASIC HYGIENE RULES

If you only have a limited amount of time, keeping the home clean is more important than keeping it tidy or dust-free. Those suffering from one type of health problem may have lower resistance to bugs, making them prone to catch anything that happens to be doing the rounds.

And then there's you, more than likely run down through the effort of being a carer, and knowing if you do get ill you won't be able to take time off. Try and prevent any germs coming into the home, by asking people who may be harbouring an infection to stay away until they're well; and observe the usual rules of hygiene in order to prevent any cross-infection between you and the person you care for.

If you're involved in any medical procedures, keep a box of surgical gloves to hand, wash surfaces regularly, and ask the health authority to give you a sharps box for the safe disposal of needles.

INCONTINENCE

Many carers find incontinence one of the hardest things to deal with. (It's not great for those it's happening too either.) Though most parents take a matter-of-fact approach to mopping up their children's accidents, loss of bladder or bowel control in adults is complicated by its associations with lack of personal hygiene, loss of control and of dignity.

If incontinence becomes a problem, the first thing to do is check whether there's any medical help available. Sometimes particular drugs or combinations of medicines can cause loss of control, and diet or an infection may also be a factor. If medical problems are ruled out the next step is to see if you can set up routines that will minimise the chances of accidents happening. Get the person you care for in the habit of going to the loo at set times, ensure the loo – or at least a commode or bottles or bedpan – are close by, and ensure they don't have a lot to drink just before bed. The third step is to use whatever aids you can to minimise its impact on you both. Your health visitor should be able to help with pads or special underwear and, if not, they're stocked by all big chemists. As they're bulky items, many companies offer a home delivery service. There are also agencies who will collect soiled items and clean up. The continence adviser should be able to give you details.

Waterproof bedding beneath the sheets will offer some protection as will lino in preference to carpet on the floor. Clothes that give quick and easy access will also help. And more sophisticated aids coming on the market now include a loo which squirts water up to clean soiled areas.

The other thing you can do is approach toileting and incontinence with a light and – if possible – humorous touch. Have you ever noticed how much children love 'poo' jokes? Somewhere en route to adulthood we seem to acquire the habit of turning up our nose at everything connected to processes which are as normal as yawning or sneezing.

If you're really struggling with what you feel, do ask for help from social services or ask the district nurse to refer you to the continence adviser. Nationally, the Continence Foundation, whose details are given in the resources section, is an excellent source of specialist advice and support.

CARRYING OUT MEDICAL PROCEDURES

Whether it's doling out tablets or emptying a catheter bag, there may be occasions where caring for someone involves being a nurse too. There are three main sources for advice. First, you can talk to the professionals: the practice or district nurse should be able to give you some training on how to carry out a range of procedures – after all, you're saving them a job. If you've time, a first aid course is another possibility. St John's Ambulance arrange courses so contact them to find out what's running in your area. Finally, you can buy or borrow a first aid manual. Again, St John's Ambulance, and the British Red Cross, are among those who publish good guides in an easy-to-use format.

The important thing to remember is that if you're not comfortable or confident about giving medical care you don't have to. You're not a trained nurse and it's perfectly OK to make your feelings clear to the doctor or hospital if you don't want to get involved. They will then have to make arrangements for a district nurse or doctor to step in.

On the other hand, if you can manage, there'll be less waiting around, fewer clashes with your own routines, and the person you're caring for knows they're in familiar hands.

If they're struggling with medicine, the most common types are available in a range of forms – not just tablets but capsules, powders, liquids, suppositories, creams or as injections. Ask the doctor if you can try an alternative form.

HELP IN GETTING AROUND

You may not want to do everything together, indeed you may regard doing chores which take you out of the house as a hint of respite. But equally, if either of you is suffering from cabin fever, frustrated by long hours at home with few distractions, then finding ways to help the person you care for to be more mobile will benefit you both.

Disability legislation means there are now few places you can't take a wheelchair and many of the large indoor shopping centres loan them to disabled visitors. Alternatively, you could try and borrow one from the hospital or Red Cross. Walking sticks, frames and wheeled walkers are other possibilities to help your loved one get around, also available from the health services or Red Cross.

HOW TO APPROACH LIFTING

It's not hard to understand why so many carers suffer from back problems. If the person you care for has mobility problems you probably find yourself struggling to help them out of bed, in and out of chairs, into the bath – tasks which no professional is allowed to do without a colleague to share the load with them.

Tackling moving and lifting tasks yourself ought to be a last resort: there are mechanical aids which can go some way to taking the strain for lifting and moving tasks and the professionals should be helping you to get them.

If you know some tasks are still going to be left to you, ask your doctor, health visitor or occupational therapist to give you some training in how to do them without injuring yourself. Some local carers centres offer training courses in moving and handling. You'll also find illustrated guidance in the first aid manuals that can be borrowed from the library.

KEEPING YOUR MINDS ACTIVE

No doubt as a carer your mind is active a lot of the time: in the middle of the night when you should be sleeping, or throughout the day, churning relentlessly onto what you've got to do next before you're halfway through the task in hand. Unfortunately, that's not the kind of brain food that acts as both a stimulant to feeling good, and a therapeutic distraction from the cares of the day.

And then there's the person you're caring for. If they are often confined to the home, cut off by circumstances from regular contact with friends and other family, time will move as achingly slowly for them as it hurtles by for you. What you both need is to give your minds a regular workout with activities you enjoy: the kind of occupations that require so much concentration you simply can't think about anything else.

Below are a few activities that other carers recommend for you to try together or apart.

STAYING ACTIVE

◆ Join a craft group or teach yourself a new craft at home.

◆ The internet is the gateway to everything from conversation and support to games, reviews, shopping and current affairs. Is there any way you can afford to get online, for them and for you?

◆ Get a tape recorder and record your loved one's story – or your own.

◆ Read aloud to each other, or borrow books on tape.

◆ Go to the cinema once a week or once a month and take it in turns to choose what you watch. If you can't get out, recreate the movies at home by making popcorn and pulling the curtains.

◆ Get some watercolours and learn to paint.

◆ Invent a recipe for a satisfying soup or a delicious dessert; or turn your favourite recipes into a cookbook for others to enjoy.

◆ Have a manicure or pedicure.

◆ Attend a lecture at the local college or museum.

◆ Create a wildlife corner in your own back garden, so you can attract birds, butterflies and other wildlife.

◆ Go to the park and feed the ducks.

◆ Visit the pet shop or garden centre to see the fish and other animals.

◆ Join a book group – or start your own.

◆ Sign up for an adult education class.

◆ Or do a home study course in anything from languages to creative writing.

◆ Join a carers support group!!

10

How Relationships are Affected

When author Sue Miller got a phone call to say the police had picked up her father, wandering confused through a strange town, her biggest challenge was how to shift her thinking: to recognise that the man who'd always looked out for her now needed her to be strong for him.

In a moving account of her father's Alzheimer's, *The Story of My Father,* Sue describes the moment when she realised she needed to switch roles with her parent. 'It became clear to me that I would need to be honest and forceful or he would never accede to me. That I would need to insist. I had never insisted on anything with my father . . . (but) we would be in charge of him now.'

Husbands and wives who suddenly find themselves caring for a partner also speak of their struggle to adjust, sometimes overnight, to a dramatically altered relationship. Whatever vows they may have made, neither had ever seriously considered the possibility that a serious accident or illness would force one of them into the role of total dependent, the other into their carer.

And what about parents who, having spent two decades nurturing their children, look forward to getting a little more of their lives back? Then find that severe mental illness, drug or alcohol dependency makes it impossible to loosen the ties of care. Their responsibilities now seem to stretch forever into the future.

Along with all the other issues caring throws up, its effects on our relationships with those we are caring for, and those around us, are among the most profound. What can you do to help yourself and others face up to them and move forward in your altered world?

CARING FOR YOUR CHILD

One of the biggest challenges facing any parent whose child's illness or disability demands more input from them than is usual is to recognise themselves as a carer who needs extra assistance and support.

Devinder's daughter Natasha developed atopic eczema, an extreme condition which meant Devinder spent hours every day bathing and creaming Natasha's burning skin, and watching her round the clock to stop her scratching herself raw. Recalls Devinder: 'The hardest bit was the sleepless nights and the pain of seeing Natasha suffer. There is an emotional side to having to watch your daughter tear herself to pieces. I couldn't work because I couldn't leave her. I didn't trust that anyone else would know how to deal with her condition and in fairness I didn't want to put them in that position.'

And yet for a long time it didn't occur to her that she was doing anything more than being the best parent she could be. Only later, when she began to recognise the eczema's impact on other areas of her life, did she acknowledge that she was a carer as well as a parent and took steps to start a support group for others in the same position.

Both different and the same – helping your child to independence
The second major hurdle you face as a parent carer is knowing how and when to give your child more independence, to allow them to develop as far as they are able and perhaps leave the family home.

Mary says it was isolation and lack of support that prevented her from seeing this until it was almost too late. The result of what she describes as 'being cocooned together for years' was that her daughter finally became violent. 'We were just stifling each other. She didn't have anywhere to go like other teenagers and say "my mum's doing my head in." When I started getting bruises I called social services.' Her daughter is now in a supported living setting but the traumatic way they parted means both continue to find the letting-go hard. 'The first three weeks she must have phoned me 80 times which was really wearing. Finally I realised if I ran to her every time we'd end up back at square one.'

As a parent carer it's important to recognise that you will still have to go through all the same struggles and stages as any other parent and child. In any family, the relationship between parent and child changes often and you need to let that happen and not confuse the difficulties of providing care with normal growing pains.

If you're struggling, do consult other carers, especially those you may meet through support groups set up specifically by and for the parents of others whose children suffer from the same illness or disability. They can help you navigate the road that leads to more independence for you both.

Managing the transition from child to adult

To add to the stress of such times, carers have found some local authorities are better than others at preparing everyone for times of transition, especially the move from school to whatever comes after. As a dependent, your child will have been the responsibility of the education service, but once they leave school they come under the care of social services. It's not unknown for this vital bit of information not to be shared with parent carers; nor for both areas in the local authority

to assume you, the child's parent, are sorting out post-school provision –
further education, training, residential care – yourself.

If your child is approaching adulthood and no one has mentioned plans
for the future, get onto them and insist you get together to discuss who is
going to do what to ensure your child doesn't fall through a gap.

CARING FOR A PARENT

As parents among you know, our children remain our children no matter
how old they get. Even when they have children of their own we're still
looking out for them. Conversely, as adults many of us remain children
around our parents, hanging onto the same patterns of behaviour, still
looking to them for support, recognition and approval. Whether we get
on with our parents or not, the deep familiarity of this first, key relationship is what makes it so challenging to relate as carer and cared-for, to
make decisions or look after the physical needs of someone who used
to do so for us. Of course there are also carers who never experienced a
sense of being looked after by their parents, which can cause them
special difficulties when the roles seem to be reversed.

At the same time it's likely you will be dealing with your parents' mixed
feelings about being in this situation at all, worry about being 'a burden',
frustration which translates into being cantankerous with you, denial, or
insistence on continuing to treat you like a child. If this is happening, it
may help to remind yourself that the difficulties in your relationship
probably existed before the caring relationship. If issues, events, feelings
from the past are unresolved between you, they are likely to be brought
into sharper focus by the amount of time you are spending together
and the alteration in your relationship. You could seek help from a
counsellor if you feel the issues are difficult enough to be getting in the
way of your carer role, or causing either of you grief.

Continue to be child and parent

For both your sakes, no matter how awkward your parent's behaviour is, resist a complete role reversal: try not to treat them like a child. This is especially challenging if they are suffering from a condition such as dementia but the trouble with treating the person you care for like a child is that they will start to behave more and more like one.

Think back to when you were a child, or to your own children. The more people did for you, the less inclined you were to do things like picking up your own clothes or making your bed yourself. At whatever level your parent is able to operate, be clear with them about their responsibilities.

Other carers say it has helped their relationship if they are able to find opportunities for their parents to continue to parent them, for instance, seeking their advice, whether it's on an important life choice or how to get Yorkshire pudding to rise. Just because you are having to dress or bathe them, it doesn't mean they don't still have something to contribute in other areas of life.

You could also experiment with ways of reinventing your relationship. After her father's diagnosis, Sue Miller recounts how much pleasure it gave her to organise for him the same kind of treats she'd enjoyed as a child: a drive out, sandwiches on a park bench, an ice cream on the way home, both of their faces alight with the joy of rediscovering sights, tasks and experiences they thought they'd left behind.

YOUNG CARERS

It's only recently that we've woken up to the fact that there are hundreds of thousands of young people taking care of a parent or siblings or both. As a young person, you may have become a carer for many reasons: because your parent's own problems – for instance some kind of dependency or mental health problem – prevent them caring fully for you and your brothers and sisters. Because they're disabled and need you to help. Or you're living with a single parent and have stepped into the gap left by the missing adult – so that sometimes you feel as if you are more of a partner to your parent than a child.

Even more than adult carers, it's important you don't try to manage alone. If you do you may miss out on the chance to develop at your own pace, it may affect your social life, your self-confidence and your education – all of which could affect your future too. It's natural to worry about your parent, and to want to protect them. But it should not be left to you to look after them alone.

Get help by involving other adults

There are a number of people you could think about talking to and asking for help:

◆ Across the country there are now young carers groups that can help you by contacting the people and organisations which are set up to support those who need care, like your parent. They can also give you the chance to meet other young carers which you may find helpful if you don't feel able to share what you're going through with mates. Being a young carer sometimes makes it hard to make friends outside the home.

◆ If there isn't a young carers group near you, or it's hard for you to contact them, the Princess Royal Trust for Carers runs a helpline especially for you. Find details in the resources section.

◆ Your local council has people trained to support carers like you. They can arrange to make an assessment of the kinds of help your family needs so that you can get on with your education, hobbies and friendships, while continuing to support your parent if you wish.

◆ Your school is another place where you can go for help. Most schools have someone whose role includes 'pastoral care' and some now have a lead teacher especially for young carers. But schools don't always know what's going on in our home lives unless we tell them. Perhaps you need to take time off school or you struggle to do your homework because of your home responsibilities. Choose a teacher you feel you can trust and tell them what's going on.

◆ Is there another adult you get on with? Perhaps the parent of one of your friends or a neighbour? You could ask them to contact a young carers group or one of the helplines for you.

Other young people in your position have come up with their own charter, setting out what we, as adults, owe to you:

YOUNG CARERS CHARTER

Children and young people have the right to:

◆ be children as well as carers

◆ get support from school and college to ensure a good education

◆ have time from caring for friendship, fun and to pursue other interests

◆ have help and support so they are not caring alone

◆ be listened to

◆ be safe

◆ be involved and given information by the other people and agencies that are involved

> ◆ be able to stop caring when they need to
>
> ◆ be helped to move on into adult life.

CARING FOR A PARTNER

Sue and John looked to have it sussed. They'd brought up two lovely children and gave up their high-pressured jobs to run a bookshop together. They were sociable, loyal to their friends, and obviously still in love after all these years. One night a friend who hadn't seen them for a while got a call out of the blue from Sue. She sounded odd and confused. John called the same friend the next day to explain she had just been diagnosed as having early-onset dementia. 'I feel better knowing what's wrong. I couldn't understand the way she'd been recently,' he said. 'But I'm scared. I'm just beginning to realise that all these years she's always been the one looking after me, taking care of everything. I don't know if I'll cope.'

For one partner to become dependent on the other is to shift a marriage or loving partnership on its axis. The very term 'partnership' conjures up equals, sharing, dreaming, building together and yet suddenly that has changed. On top of dealing with day-to-day care you may be having to come to terms with the loss of the future you planned, with the loss of a friend, a sexual companion, a co-parent.

This is a huge amount of loss to contemplate and to do so alone may be more than most of us can handle. A relationship counselling agency such as Relate can give you help in recognising what has changed and in dealing with all the difficult feelings that surround it. Depending on your partner's condition, they may be able to work with you both to find out what you can still be to each other, despite your changed circumstances.

Dealing with the effects on your sex life

In *The Selfish Pig's Guide to Caring* Hugh Marriott describes the effect being a carer has on our sex lives as one of the great unspoken secrets. So many of us come at sex through our feelings, and if those change, our need or desire for sex may be altered too.

Having to perform intimate tasks for your partner may well affect the way you feel about them, especially if there are times when you feel more like a parent or brother or sister to them. Sexual desire may start to feel inappropriate, even distasteful. Or it may be that dealing with all the other emotions caring brings up, as well as its physical demands, simply leaves you no energy to want sex.

Your feelings are perfectly reasonable and you need to respect them. But that may be easier said than done if the person you're caring for still wants a sexual relationship with you. Their condition may not have affected their sex drive, indeed it may have heightened it. At the same time their feelings of dependency may lead them to see sex as a way of reassuring themselves that you continue to love them.

Here again, you should seek help from a relationship counsellor, who may refer you to a psychosexual counsellor. They are trained to help you look at such difficult feelings in a 'safe' environment and will be neither judgemental nor shocked. They'll have encountered people who feel the way you do many times before, help you work out if there are ways of meeting some of your and your partner's needs, and assist you to live with the feelings you have.

And while we're on the subject of sex

And then there is the possibility that though you've lost sexual feeling for your partner, you haven't lost desire altogether. Particularly if you are still relatively young when you become your partner's carer, the fear that you may have to live for years or even the rest of your life without sex can add considerably to the stress you are already under. Only you know how you feel about the notion of finding other ways to have your sexual needs met. Your views may prohibit you seeking sexual relations outside of your relationship – and so might your timetable!

But if sex *is* important to you then you need to recognise that it contributes significantly to your physical and emotional well-being. And since you cannot be the best carer you can be if your own needs are being denied, then your usual notions of what is appropriate behaviour may no longer fit in this new world you find yourself in.

HOW CARING CAN AFFECT THOSE AT HOME

Inevitably, if one member of the family requires more from you, others (including you) will end up with less. There are only 24 hours – even in a carer's day. You may not be in a position to do much about this but being aware of it and acknowledging it is important for everyone. For instance, don't assume that other family members, especially children, will just naturally understand why they can't have more of your time and attention. Understand their jealousy or resentment if that's what they are feeling and remind them and yourself that those feelings are pretty normal in households without any illness or disability. Every child wants to be the centre of its parents' life.

Regular check-in time will give them a chance to express what they are feeling: this really is a case where the quality of the time you are able to give them is worth more than its quantity. At the same time watch yourself for any signs that you are leaning more than you should be on them, making them *your* carers. There is a big difference between asking them to do their fair share of chores, contributing to the household, and looking to them for emotional support. However much of a carer you are, you remain their parent and should be looking to other adults for the support you need.

If you live with a partner, that relationship is going to need your attention too. It may be that you're never in the same room, either because you're taking it in turns to care, or because you are carrying the load as a carer while practicalities such as the need for an income or to care for others in the house mean your partner is always fully occupied with their duties. You're like trains on parallel tracks, watching each other hurtle along at speed but never close enough or slow enough to touch.

Adversity can sometimes bring people closer together. For every carer who regrets the way a marriage or special relationship was damaged by the amount of energy they had to put into caring, there is another for whom their partner proved an anchor, the solidity at the core of their lives.

The thing to keep reminding yourself is that while the day-to-day health of your relationship may be affected by your carer role, its strength depends on precisely the same things as any other loving relationship, including all those in which no one is a carer: your commitment to each other and to making it work, to sharing yourselves and your feelings, to being honest with each other, and to supporting and being supported by each other.

HOW YOUR RELATIONSHIPS WITH OTHER RELATIVES MAY BE AFFECTED

One of the saddest things about becoming carer to her mother was that it estranged Lizzie from her sister Anne. When their mother could no longer cope with living alone it was Lizzie who was the nearest. Rather than move her into residential care, Lizzie decided she'd sell her house and move in with their mother so she could stay in her own home.

Says Lizzie: 'Anne and I spoke about it and I thought she was OK with the decision. It turns out she wasn't. She thought I was trying to get hold of mum's money and property for myself. That hurt me more than anything because as far as I was concerned I'd put my life on hold to help mum. Anne never lifted a finger, not really. Perhaps I should have told her I was feeling dumped on by her and she might have been able to be honest about her worries. We haven't spoken since mum died.'

Lizzie and Anne's broken relationship is a salutary lesson in the importance of frequent and honest communication among all those who have a stake in your caring role.

It may seem unfair that as well as being a carer you're having to make the running in talking to other relatives – as if you didn't have enough to do. There are certainly plenty of cases where carers feel, quite rightly, that other family members aren't doing enough; that they have literally been left 'holding the baby' because they live nearest, or aren't working, or have fewer 'family' responsibilities.

The only way to know what is going on is to talk and listen in equal measure to each other. It's possible other family members might want to do more but feel shut out by the closeness of your relationship with their loved one. Maybe there are times when, without realising it, you make it hard for them to get involved because keeping control is your way of coping.

Take another look at the section in this book on assertiveness (see Chapter 4), which should help you be honest and clear with your relatives without anger or other negative feelings getting in the way. And have a think about the items in the checklist below which may be affecting all of your relationships.

RELATIONSHIP CHECKLIST

Whether being a carer makes or breaks your other relationships is down to everyone:

◆ Share as much of the practical care as you can. It's a way of reinforcing that you are a family and have responsibility for each other.

◆ Are you sure you're not excluding them? When we're under pressure we often feel it's quicker and easier to do things ourselves. Ask them if they ever feel as if you're cutting them out.

◆ Organise regular family meetings to keep everyone in touch.

◆ Recognise that other people make different choices and you can't change them. Your siblings, friends or family may be well aware of what you are doing as a carer but choose not to get involved. If that's the case it's probably best to let go of your expectations to avoid being hurt by feelings of let-down and resentment.

◆ Be aware that family issues, roles and resentments from the past may be revived by this new, stressful situation. Try to avoid getting 'hooked in' to the past.

◆ Don't try and be a counsellor for everyone. As the main carer, you may feel pressured by others into acting as a counsellor for them. But you can't take on everyone's problems – and they shouldn't expect you to.

◆ Don't be defined by your carer role. You are so much more.

CHANGING RELATIONSHIPS: WHAT OTHER CARERS SAY

'At some stage I realised the relationship had changed from being lovers to me being her carer. I loved her dearly. I never stopped, but the sexual side just petered out. The changes in our relationship were like summer going into autumn, but we didn't ever discuss it.' **Tony**

'I think the worst thing for me was that mum and I never got on when I was a kid. It was always my brother this, my brother that, and I resented it. I thought why should I have to look after you? You hated me when I was a kid and now I'm lumbered.' **Linda**

'I've been looking after my father's physical needs for some time now and I can see it bothers him that I have to do it. So I've started to talk to him about some of my problems, things going on in my life and given him a chance to offer his take on them. Not only is his advice often spot-on, it makes him feel we have a more equal relationship. He's still my dad.' **Bill**

'When I was 15 dad left. He told me I was responsible for everyone and I've been locked into the family ever since. I'm still more like a mother to my sisters. Recently I asked my dad "why did you say that?" and he said "because I knew you'd be able to sort it out".' **Teresa**

'My brother said move up here and I'll help you out. He used to pop in from work for 15 minutes three times a week. That was it, that was his bit. For a carer, actions always speak louder than words. We've hardly spoken since mum died.' **Janet**

11

So, How Are You Feeling?

One of the toughest things about caring for my uncle was knowing what to do with some of the things I was feeling: resentment about having to park every other important thing in my own life in order to care for him; anger that he assumed my time was his and would continue to be; frustration that my plans for life were on hold; guilt, that I felt all these things when it was he who was dying.

No matter what your motivations for being a carer, what circumstances brought you to this point, it's likely that as well as dealing with daily life you are having to cope with a whole range of difficult feelings.

And, if you're like most of us, your way of coping is probably by pretending those feelings aren't even there, suppressing them because:

◆ you are ashamed of them – your thoughts run something like, 'it's them who is suffering, I'm the lucky one. I have no right to feel the way I do'

◆ you're scared – if you allow such powerful feelings any space in your life you fear they'll overwhelm you and tip you over the edge

◆ you believe they're a sign of weakness, or your fault – if you could just be a better person or love the person you care for more you wouldn't be feeling this way, would you?

Consider this. If the six million other carers out there didn't feel those same horrible emotions as you sometimes, there wouldn't need to be 800 carer support groups throughout the UK. No matter what it is you're feeling, you have good reasons to do so. No matter how unacceptable some of those emotions are to you, there are hundreds of thousands of others who feel exactly the same way. The aim of this section is to help you recognise and live with those feelings.

WHOSE LIFE IS IT ANYWAY? FEELINGS OF LOSS

Loss is something most of us know about. At some point in our lives someone we care about has died and we expect to feel sadness that they have gone from our lives. When someone we know is bereaved, we treat them with compassion and gentleness.

Life as a carer is like going through a series of bereavements. First there are the practical losses you're suffering: the hours in your day or week that are no longer available to you, the loss of income, giving up your job perhaps, losing your privacy, the end of your social life, the time to see friends. For those of you caring for dementia sufferers there may in addition be the 'loss' of your loved one; they are still there but no longer recognisable.

And then there is the loss of your plans for your own life. Perhaps they weren't huge: you just wanted to take up gardening or learn to use a computer. Perhaps they were major schemes: marriage and children, a career change, backpacking round the world. Perhaps they were dreams you shared with the one who is now dependent on you: instead of a peaceful retirement you are left contemplating a lonely future of looking after someone who you thought would be your soulmate.

Whether or not you're able to articulate what you want from life as clearly as that, do recognise that somewhere along the line you are having to adjust your own dreams to fit the reality of your life now as a carer. You may find yourself asking 'whose life is it anyway?' like James, caring for his mother, who says: 'That's what it comes down to for me. I'm living the life of a 92-year-old woman.'

Treat yourself with the same compassion and gentleness as you would anyone who is having to come to terms with loss on this scale. You are suffering from a major bereavement – except that unlike the bereavement that follows death, you have to face your loss anew each day.

Bereavement counsellors talk of going through stages of loss, from sadness, anger, guilt, depression, even despair, towards recovery. Because your bereavement is continuing, you may experience any or all of those feelings at any time without the knowledge that those strong emotions will eventually pass, to be replaced by more manageable feelings.

FEELINGS OF ANGER

Anger may be directed at ourselves, at the person we are caring for, and at the world in general. Just as when we were children we reacted angrily to things we thought were unfair, we're angry that life has thrown us this one. If the person you're caring for is suffering, physically or emotionally, that may add to your rage. You'd take the hurt away from them if you could, and the fact that you can't, your impotence, adds fuel to the angry fires inside. And then there is the 'unacceptable' face of anger, what we sometimes feel about the person we are supposed to be taking care of. Sometimes their behaviour makes us angry. That's life: very few of us are saints. Sometimes something else causes the anger but we take it out on those we love: that's normal too.

The trouble is that in a care situation anger doesn't feel safe. We may not want to express it to the person we're caring for because we know they're vulnerable. But trying to keep a lid on it really is like someone trying to contain a volcanic crater with a plug. The explosion will come and when it does, its effects could be a great deal more damaging for you – or the person you're caring for.

A strategy for dealing with anger

You need to deal with the pinches before you get to the crunch, to learn to recognise when you are feeling angry and leave the room. Even if you are worried about leaving your loved one, it's safer for you both if you tell them you are leaving the room for 10 minutes and walk away from the situation. Once you have left, take some deep breaths to bring your adrenaline levels down. Then, discharge your anger. This is the lava erupting, but doing so with you in control of when it happens and how it is channelled. There are a number of ways you can do this:

◆ make your own punchbag from old clothes stuffed into a sack and suspended from a joist in the garage

◆ buy loads of old china from a car boot sale so each time your feelings reach boiling point you can hurl a plate in the garden

◆ find a private place and scream, loud and long

◆ take a tennis racket to a cushion or pillow

◆ go for a power walk round the garden.

You will feel better when you have done something physical to release your feelings and that's the time to spend a few moments assessing the situation. What's caused your anger: a build-up of tensions or stresses; a single remark or incident? And do you need to do anything about it: tackle the cause, review the situation that's causing such difficult feelings, get more help for you? If the anger is telling you something important, those moments after you've discharged it are vital for your emotional and physical health.

FACING UP TO OTHER DIFFICULT FEELINGS

Feelings of resentment

If the one you're caring for doesn't seem to appreciate what you're doing for them you may well feel resentful. Or you may resent those you feel aren't helping out as much as they could: other members of your family or the professionals. You may, in a generalised way, resent those who appear to be getting on with their lives without having the caring responsibilities that you do: colleagues, friends, neighbours . . . the rest of the world. Of course you know in your head that they probably have their own trials and tribulations but in your heart a little voice sometimes hisses 'it's alright for them'.

Resentment is a nasty emotion because rather than exploding it seeps into your life, your thoughts, your tone, and it's you that is most affected. Imagine you were forced to wear dark sunglasses so even on a glorious summer's day, or looking at a golden sunset, all you can see are shades of grey. Resentment is like that. It stops you seeing beauty or pleasure or even facing each new day with a clear pair of eyes.

If your resentment stems from people not pulling their weight then tell them what you feel, and do so assertively rather than resentfully. Then park the rest: the stuff you can't do anything about because you're the one it's hurting. It's your world turning grey.

Feelings of guilt

And then the next moment, being the kind of person you are, you're feeling guilty for having felt anything negative at all. Every carer I have ever spoken to has felt guilty about something. Guilty that they're not doing enough for their loved ones, or enough of the right thing. Guilty that the others in their lives – partners, children, friends – are not getting enough attention. Guilty that they're not doing their work as well as they ought to be because of everything else that's going on. And – in a horrible Catch 22 – guilty that these feelings are sometimes being expressed in anger or resentment around their loved ones, which makes them feel even more guilty.

Let's face it, no matter how much we do for our loved ones, no matter how many somersaults we turn trying to do the right thing by everyone, we feel it will never be enough. Actually it is. No one can do more than their best. You can't do more than your best and you're already doing that. Forgive yourself. Your best is enough.

Feelings of loneliness and isolation

As a carer you may be largely housebound and feel utterly cut off and under-stimulated. Alternatively you may be the embodiment of the saying that you can feel alone in a crowd: your life could hardly be busier and yet you feel completely isolated. In either case these feelings are likely to stem from the sense that no one understands your position. You're not getting help and everything is left to you. You are, in addition, experiencing all these difficult emotions and feel you can't share them with anyone because you think they're unacceptable.

Feelings of loneliness may also stem from loss. Especially if you are caring for a partner, you may no longer have the person you used to share everything with. You don't have time to share your feelings with friends, like you used to, and in any case, who'd be interested? It's not as if being a carer is exciting and gives you something to talk about!

Loneliness is less about being alone than about feeling unseen and unvalued – which is why you should look at the sections in this book on what other carers say. And think about finding other carers through a carers centre or one of the organisations listed in the resources section. You really are only one phone call or a few clicks of the computer mouse away from talking to someone who knows exactly how you feel.

ACCEPTING THE WAY YOU FEEL

Those are just a few of the tough feelings you may be experiencing. Other carers speak of feeling hopeless, depressed, frustrated, furious, sad and desperate. These are huge emotions. Any one of them would be enough to overwhelm you sometimes. No wonder when someone does ask how you're doing you say 'fine'. The most important thing for you to understand is that everything you are feeling *is* fine. You *cannot* choose or control what you feel, only what you do with those feelings.

Think of those outtake shows where someone slips over into the water. Your first reaction is laughter, even if the part of you that knows laughing is wrong in case someone was hurt quickly gets control of your instinctive response.

There is a part of many of us that refuses to believe that we can't control our feelings: that thinks if only we try harder, or were better people, we would never feel angry or bitter, never snap at those we love. But aren't you already trying? Aren't you someone who is doing the best job they can in difficult circumstances?

Instead of fighting yourself and your feelings, recognise them for what they are: your deepest self telling you how it is, what effect caring is having on you.

LISTENING TO YOUR FEELINGS

Once you stop fighting your feelings and acknowledge them you can work out whether you need to act on them. If you think any of them is in danger of running out of control, if they seem unmanageable or out or proportion to what's going on, if you think there is a chance of you lashing out at someone else, you have reached a point where you need to get support. In the same way that animals instinctively react to a looming storm by seeking shelter, long before there is any obvious sign of the danger to come, our feelings are our early warning systems. Turn to the sections on sharing care and getting support for you (Chapters 12 and 13) for advice on where to get help right now.

On the other hand, you may find allowing yourself to acknowledge and accept your feelings – and forgiving yourself for having them – takes away some of their power to damage you. The energy that you've been diverting into resisting those difficult emotions, keeping the lid on them, is now available for you to direct into more positive areas of your life.

Copy or cut out the Carer's Creed on the next page and stick it beside your bed so you can look at it every morning before the day starts and every night when the day is done.

CARER'S CREED

◆ Whatever I feel able to do is enough.

◆ Things don't have to be perfect: I can drop my standards.

◆ I will treat myself with the same gentleness and understanding that I would another carer.

◆ Negative feelings don't make me a bad person; they mean I'm in a bad situation.

◆ I'm not a saint: I will not let other people's expectations get in the way of me doing the best I can.

◆ From now on I will work out what I can and can't change and stop worrying about everything in the 'can't' column.

WHAT TO DO IF YOU'RE SUFFERING FROM STRESS OR DEPRESSION

Sometimes when we try to suppress our feelings for a long time they damage us and lead to serious conditions such as stress and depression. There are many reasons why, as a carer, you may be suffering from stress: you're juggling so many conflicting demands; you're worried about money; being a carer is physically exhausting; you don't know how long the situation will go on for; and you feel out of control. The important thing is to know when stress is producing symptoms which could cause you worse harm. And to get support from your doctor, or from one of the sources we'll look at in the next section on getting help for you.

How to recognise stress

Stress expresses itself in a huge number of different ways. Take a look at the list below. If you tick more than two or three of these symptoms you've probably reached the stage of needing to make some changes, seek support or get medical help before you get more sick.

❑ You wake in the night worrying and find it impossible to switch off.

❑ You have real trouble getting to sleep in the first place.

❑ You're drinking more alcohol, smoking more cigarettes or eating more of the wrong foods than is good for you.

❑ You get tearful at what seem to be small things.

❑ People and situations irritate you far more than they used to.

❑ Your mood sometimes swings wildly but your highs and lows are not necessarily related to what's going on.

❑ You suffer from headaches, high blood pressure, sickness, loss of appetite, muscular twitches, rashes.

❑ You feel exhausted all the time.

❑ You feel stretched to breaking point.

❑ You've stopped enjoying things that used to give you pleasure.

❑ You catch every virus that is going around.

How to recognise depression

Depression is a medical condition. It may have been triggered by some of the factors we've discussed, by physical and emotional overload as a result of being a carer. But it's medical help you need first to prevent your condition getting worse and even affecting your ability to go on caring.

Though seeking support with your caring role and for yourself will help in time, one of the insidious symptoms of depression is its power to rob you of the energy, will and confidence to take such action. So see your doctor first, and only when you're feeling stronger look at the next chapter and how you can build enough support into your life as a carer to try and prevent depression returning.

Among the signs that you may be suffering from depression are:

❑ You feel sad, lonely and anxious all the time.

❑ You're not sure what gets you up in the morning.

❑ You feel angry with everyone.

❑ No matter what you do, you feel it's not enough.

❑ The slightest demand sends you screaming into the corner.

❑ You can't remember when you last laughed.

❑ You can't seem to make a decision about anything.

❑ Sometimes you think it would be easier to die.

❑ You have suicidal thoughts.

DIFFICULT FEELINGS: WHAT OTHER CARERS SAY

'I feel guilty. Mum thinks I'm doing too much but my big failing is I'm not always as patient as I should be. When I'm stressed out I don't do things as well as I might. And then that makes mum feel like she's a burden.' **Ros**

'I'm not proud of this but when I get home really tired and my son's room's in a mess I shout at him and tell him he's no good. And of course it's not really him I'm angry with at all but this whole, awful situation. The trouble is, once I've said those things the damage is done and I feel even worse.' **Jill**

'I've got no regrets except that I used to lose my rag occasionally. I think it was sheer frustration. One day she'd taken herself off to the toilet somehow but then she'd slipped and there was mess all over the floor. I just lost it. I turned and walked out for ten minutes. I still think about that.' **Tony**

'Mum used to sit in the kitchen all the time and I'd sit with her where I could see the front door. It's got these wooden bars: they were like prison bars for me.' **Janet**

12

Sharing the Caring Role

For years I resisted the idea of paying a cleaner to give my home a basic once-over each week. I should be able to fit it in somehow, I thought, and then another week would go by and as I rushed around trying to be a working single parent and carer I'd feel I was failing badly because we were going home to a dirty house.

The terms 'superwoman' and 'superman' are not compliments but burdens: trying to live up to them is simply another load on our backs. The sooner we allow ourselves to at least consider the possibility that we could share some of the load, the better it will be for both our physical and emotional health. If you haven't yet asked for a carer assessment, it's time to reconsider whether you should, and to start exploring all the other ways in which you could get help carrying the weight of your caring responsibilities.

FACING UP TO THE BARRIERS TO SHARING CARE

Cooking, cleaning, shopping, gardening, even sitting, are just a few of the jobs you could share with professionals, other family members, neighbours or friends. A carer assessment may provide for some of those services in the care plan. But even if it doesn't it's worth weighing up the benefits to you both of getting help with the day-to-day work. You're almost certainly not flush with cash but if you know there is enough money to just about get by and it's the principle of paying that is holding you back, remind yourself that (a) it's to buy such support services that benefits are paid, and (b) that what the money's actually buying is time for you – time being the one thing that is priceless.

If the kitty truly is empty and social services has failed to come up with much in the way of a care package, then it's time to take up any of the offers of help you get from the unpaid workforce of relatives, friends and neighbours. Knowing what's involved in being a carer you may feel reluctant to involve other people but you're not asking them to do what you do. You're only responding positively to their offers to take a tiny part of the load off your shoulders.

And while you're still in full control of your loved one's care, it's surprising how small amounts of help add up. If you're used to only getting one hour to yourself a day (and that will seem generous to some carers) then an extra two or three hours' help a week is a significant improvement.

OVERCOMING THEIR OBJECTIONS

Another objection that carers come up with is that the person they're caring for won't allow anyone else to be involved. That's OK if you really are superhuman and plan never to get ill, tired, fretful, or in any way temporarily unable to be a carer. But you're not. And what will happen if you don't get help is that you'll get ill and they'll have to put up with other carers whether they like it or not.

I'm not underestimating how huge a task it can be to force the issue. This is one of those situations many carers name as their biggest challenge. But the way you choose to handle it is about showing love and compassion for you both. If you need to, you're allowed to share the responsibility by saying your doctor's ordered you to take a rest (whether or not you've actually sought medical advice). Or to claim you need a few days to deal with an emergency elsewhere. Whatever it takes.

Or you can choose to be honest and tell them that if you don't get more help and the occasional break you're worried you won't be able to go on caring. It may not be ideal – but they'll survive and be looked after. What's more, in a relationship that is probably one-sided, agreeing to something that will help you is one way in which they can give you some care back.

Sometimes it's change people are scared of and once they get used to a professional carer coming in, or to spending a week once or twice a year in respite care, they may welcome the break, and the new faces, as much as you do. After all, you may be the most fascinating person in the world but if you're the only one the person you care for gets to see and talk to every day that fascination may get a little jaded.

BRINGING HELP IN

Sitting service

Sitters can stand in for you, keep the person you're caring for company, ensure they're safe, and carry out basic care tasks such as preparing food.

If your relatives aren't pulling their weight, you could suggest they set aside two or three hours once a week or even once a month to come and sit with the person you care for. (But remember, if they don't want to you won't be able to make them so let it go.) Alternatively, see if you can get regular sitting sessions written into the care plan as essential respite time for you.

If you want to go it alone you can still contact social services to see if they keep a list of people registered for sitting. The alternative is to go through an agency, which is expensive, but gives you the security of knowing the sitter has been checked. And you have a little more freedom to try out a few sitters until you find one that really hits it off with your loved one.

Private nurse

Before you go down this route do check to see if you can get nursing help through the doctor's surgery from a district nurse, or as part of the care plan. You don't have to perform nursing tasks if you'd rather not. But depending on the level of care the person you look after needs, there may be situations when bringing in a private nurse frees you up significantly.

Private nurses are fully trained and would expect to tackle a great deal more than a sitter, for instance dealing with catheters, changing drips, administering oxygen, as well as more fundamental care tasks such as feeding or giving a bath.

If you're setting up something by yourself you'll find nursing agencies listed in the telephone yellow pages. These supply staff whose qualifications and references have been checked and who can provide cover day or night, or for shorter sessions in between.

Home help

Home helps are usually employed to look after the household rather than the person you're caring for, though they often end up doing more simply because life doesn't fit into neat boxes. Again, social services may arrange this for you – or at least contribute towards it – as part of the care plan. If not, do consider whether paying someone to come in and clean, tidy, wash, iron, cook, wash up, would pay you back in savings in time and energy.

If you're handling recruitment yourself, the UK Homecare Association, whose contact details are in the resources section at the back of this guide, is a good place to start.

As with bringing in any paid help, your instincts are a good guide to whether the person will be a good fit with your loved one. But always ask for references and, if possible, phone rather than write to check them out. People are increasingly wary of putting anything prejudicial on paper: you'll discover much more, good or bad, if you're able to explain what the person will be doing and ask the referee to comment verbally on their suitability and reliability. And always suggest a trial period so that you can assess with the person being cared for whether they feel safe and good around the newcomer.

CARE OPTIONS OUTSIDE THE HOME

Day centres

Day centres are wonderful places, geared to providing interest, activity and support for people of varying ages and a range of conditions, depending on their own specialty. Some are run by the social services or education departments of your local council, some by charities such as the Red Cross and Age Concern, and some by private companies. However, both charity and private day centres are often under contract to provide places for clients referred to them by the professionals within social services. Many of them also offer transport to and from the centre.

The best way in is a referral from social services or the doctor. But arranging for your loved one to be a day client at a private residential home is also possible if you can afford it. There's more on residential care in Chapter 15.

If your loved one has cancer they may qualify to attend a day centre at a local hospice. Like other centres, these are activity based, offering everything from occupational therapy, arts and crafts to massage and hairdressing.

Even one day a week can break things up for you both, and attending regularly brings a new circle of carers and companions into their life.

Holidays

A number of voluntary organisations offer holiday packages, either for the person you care for by themselves, or for you to go together. If you're looking for a break, together or from each other, your starting point could be Tourism for All (see the resources section), which provides information about affordable holidays with accommodation and transport suited to those who are ill or disabled. Some will require you to accompany the person you care for, but provide plenty of support to ensure you get a bit of a break too. Others will act as stand-in carers, with trained staff taking over your caring role for a week or two.

Local authorities may also have funds to pay for respite for the one you care for, freeing you up, or to pay directly for a holiday for you. Some carers centres also have funds to enable carers to have a holiday.

Another source of information may be those charities set up to support people with specific conditions, and their carers. Mencap, for instance, organises holidays for unaccompanied children and adults and publishes a holiday accommodation guide to places where people with a learning disability are welcome.

If you do arrange a holiday for the person you're caring for, you may be tempted to simply curl up and stay home while they're away. That's fine, unless you discover you're so used to being frantically busy you end up using the time to catch up on other jobs. Don't! If there's one certainty in life it is that no matter how much you do, the jobs are never complete. It will do you so much more good to have a complete rest. If you must be busy, find some sort of relaxing activity instead: get out, visit a local museum or gallery, arrange to have coffee with friends.

And do consider taking a holiday yourself. Don't you deserve to have someone preparing and clearing up after your meals, not even to have to make your own bed if you don't want to? Tourism for All can recommend accommodation where carers are welcome alone.

Respite care

It's worth considering all of the options we've just run through when you need some respite. You may have practical reasons for wanting time out from caring: wanting to take your children on holiday, or to meet some other important commitment in your life. Or you may need respite to give yourself a physical and mental break from caring, a chance to recharge your batteries. Among those organisations that may help you get a break is Crossroads, which runs schemes in many parts of England and Wales offering help in the home. See the resources section for details.

Respite outside the home is usually provided in a residential care setting, though holidays and hospice care are also options, depending on the condition of the person you care for.

We'll look at residential care in more detail in Chapter 15, but you may find, even as a respite option, that the person you care for resists the idea. They may fear unfamiliar surroundings and routines or believe that going to spend two weeks in a residential home is the thin end of the wedge, a way of easing them into residential care permanently. If that's the case your best option may be to bring in a nurse or sitter and go away yourself.

Your alternative is to be completely honest. Tell the social worker or doctor that you are desperate for a break and that without it, you're in danger of getting ill which will mean they'll have to take over the entire caring role. Be upfront with the person you're caring for. They may not like it but you have to recharge your batteries so you can return and be there for them again. Ask them to treat it as much as they can as a holiday for them too.

SHARING CARE: WHAT OTHER CARERS SAY

'It became obvious mum wasn't managing to look after the house so after we went in and did a cleaning blitz we persuaded her she needed a home help, which she still has. The next thing was food. I was spending two or three hours there every evening cooking dinner. Now we've found someone to come in to do dinner four times a week which means I get home earlier those evenings. It's paid for out of mum's attendance allowance.' **Ros**

'I thought dad would be upset when the health visitor said she'd try and get him a few days at the hospice but he used to look forward to those days so much. They'd offer him a bath if he wanted, which was wonderful because he could only manage a shower at home. And before they served lunch – which was all properly set out with tablecloths and flowers on the table – they always offered him a glass of sherry. He said it was like going to dinner in a hotel.' **Jane**

'It got to the stage where I thought oh, I wish you weren't my mother. I would feel like pulling my hair out and then I'd think I have to get out, she's doing my head in. And I'd send my husband or the kids over instead and then feel really guilty, guilty that I didn't show her I loved her as much as I should have done.'
Linda

13

Getting Support for You

With just about everything you do in life, from sewing to speaking Swahili, the more you do it, the better you get. Except caring. You may well get better at it in the sense of being more able to juggle all the competing demands or change a bandage more quickly. But far from getting easier, most carers find it gets harder with each passing day.

The reason is not hard to fathom. Most of us are capable of switching up a gear when circumstances demand it, when we're in a hurry to get somewhere for instance. But if you sit for too long in the fast lane you start to get tired and the fuel begins to run low. To add to your stress you may not even know how long the journey's going to be.

That's why they invented service areas, to give you a rest, a chance to refuel and service the vehicle, and if necessary get some help planning the rest of the route. There are 'service areas' for carers too, but unlike those you'll find on the motorway they're not always easy to spot. Nor will you see signposts telling you 'tiredness kills – take a break'.

FINDING AND ASKING FOR HELP

In the last chapter we looked at some of your choices for sharing the caring. This chapter is about getting help for *you* from a range of informal sources, whether you need a chat, the company of people who understand, tips and advice, or a more sustained programme of counselling or emotional support.

Before we look at useful sources of support try the quiz below to see how easy you find it to ask for help. Be sure to answer the questions honestly: this is for your benefit, no one else's.

How easy do you find it to ask for help?

1. **You're meeting a friend outside the Post Office in a town you've not visited before and you're already 10 minutes late. Do you:**
   a) ring his mobile, apologise for being late and ask him for directions
   b) head for the town centre and, when you haven't found the Post Office after a few minutes, stop someone to ask
   c) weave your way around the town centre until you spot the sign, even though you're now 20 minutes overdue?

2. **At the supermarket when the cashier asks if you need any help packing do you:**
   a) say 'yes please'– four hands are obviously better than two
   b) decline, unless there's already someone standing there – you wouldn't want to upset them
   c) always say 'no' – no one else packs the way you like it done?

3. **You bump into a neighbour who says they haven't seen you for a while and asks how you are. Do you**
   a) admit that you've been tied up caring for a loved one and that though you want to do it you are finding it a struggle
   b) agree you've not been home much lately then ask them how they are
   c) smile and say 'I'm fine thank you'?

4. **Your busiest friend is organising a surprise birthday party for her husband but when she phones to invite you and hears about your life she says 'let me know if there's anything I can do to help.' Do you**
a) thank her and suggest that after the party you'll call her to discuss how she can help
b) say 'oh you've got far too much on your plate' but decide if she disagrees or offers again you might find a job for her to do
c) change the subject back to the party – offering to help is just something people do to be polite; they don't really mean it?

5. **A social worker comes to see you and suggests you need a break. She says she'll arrange respite care for your loved one but after three weeks you've not heard anything. Do you**
a) phone her on her direct line to ask whether she has managed to set something up
b) assume that no news is bad news – if she'd been able to do something you would have heard by now
c) shrug: it's what you expected; they never seem able to deliver what they say they will?

Mostly (a)s: Well done. Even if you'd rather manage alone you've learned how to ask for help and recognise your own limitations. The chances are you've already made efforts to get yourself support in your caring role. But take a look at the suggestions below to see if there's any more help you could access.

Mostly (b)s: You seem to recognise that you need help but your sensitivity to everyone else's feelings is preventing you being direct about your needs. Remember, carers need care too. Being able to ask for help is a sign of strength, not weakness.

Mostly (c)s: Poor you. It sounds as if any attempts you've made to get help have ended in disappointment and you'd rather not ask at all than have to deal with being let down again. It will take a lot of courage to change your attitude and look for help. You could start gently by accepting any offers that come your way, and by reminding yourself the best-tuned engine will judder to a halt when it runs out of fuel.

If your answers were mainly (b)s and (c)s, it may help to keep reminding yourself of the following.

TIPS

◆ It's not personal – if someone turns you down or agrees to help and then doesn't deliver, it's down to them, nothing to do with you. Tell yourself it's not intended to hurt you, remember not to ask them again, and let it go.

◆ A useful way of expressing your need for help is to agree with whoever you're asking that they give you permission to ask if you give them permission to say no. That will help you both be honest.

◆ Learn to distinguish doers from sayers. As the saying goes, if you want something done, ask a busy person.

◆ Don't underestimate the value of small acts of helping. Someone watering the garden once a week frees up 15 minutes you could spend on a phone call to a friend or having an afternoon nap.

◆ Don't feel guilty. Think for a moment about how you feel when you're able to help someone, even if it's only someone stopping you in the street and asking for directions. Most of us get a gentle glow from knowing we're being helpful. Don't deprive others of that!

JOINING A CARERS CENTRE OR SUPPORT GROUP

Actions don't always speak louder than words. Practical help is wonderful, but so too is sitting down with someone and knowing that every word you say will be not just understood but accepted in the right spirit. To the rest of the world you may hesitate to admit how truly bad it sometimes gets. But among other carers, and those who support them, you know everything you say is safe.

To find a centre in your area call the local library, ask at your doctor's surgery, or contact one of the national carer organisations listed in the resources section. If that doesn't yield anything you could always think about starting up your own support group!

Yes, I know you're already tearingly busy but think about what you'll get from a support group:

◆ *empathy* – the comfort of being with people who know what you're going through even if you don't feel like talking about it

◆ *honesty* – to be and to share yourself with no one sitting in judgement

◆ *advice* – if you want it from those who have been there, done that, and got a wardrobe full of t-shirts

◆ *humour* – it's possible that only with other carers will you find relief in laughing about the impossible, the awful, and the ridiculous

◆ *hope* – listening to other people's problems can take some of the sting out of yours, and offer solutions to problems you thought had no answer.

Apart from contact with other carers, centres offer a range of other support services, for instance, one group has arranged for former carers to ring current carers every morning, just to make sure that every single day they have someone they can offload to if they wish: someone caring about them. Other groups offer hand or neck massage to carers, problem-solving such as equipping carers with a mobile phone so they can stay in touch while they're out, or, if they're housebound, a home computer so they can contact other carers online.

GETTING CONNECTED

These days not all networks are physical. The advent of the internet has made possible the creation of a myriad of new networks reflecting people's needs and interests – and naturally that includes carers.

If your caring responsibilities mean you are often housebound, do consider what help you could get online. All of the major carers' organisations have websites where you'll find loads of useful information and links. And being the internet of course, you are not limited to this country. You can drop in on support groups anywhere around the globe if you fancy stretching your horizons.

You'll find that many of these groups have chat rooms, or email groups, where you are free to sound off, compare notes with others, share your experiences, and ask others in a similar situation for tips and solutions to problems you may have.

For many carers, online means 'lifeline'. If you think it would make a difference to you, but buying a computer is beyond you financially, it's well worth looking at whether you could get a grant from a charity, or even from social services, to help you get connected. Often when big companies upgrade their equipment they pass redundant – but still perfectly functional – computers to local charities who, in turn, distribute them to those in most need.

Another route, if you are able to leave the house occasionally, is the library service. Most libraries now have public computers offering free internet access.

One more thing you will find online are a number of stroppy carers – and that's good news. These are folk who sometimes feel the same anger, frustration and despair as the rest of us but have found that channelling those emotions into campaigning for a better deal for carers is an excellent outlet for their strong feelings.

If there are times when you find yourself spitting with fury about some professional's inability to return a phone call, about the abysmal level of funding with which social services is expected to support carers, or about the pittance carer's allowance represents, try venting your spleen in an email to your MP, to the PM, or to the government department where these decisions are made. It can be as therapeutic as locking yourself in the loo and screaming at the top of your voice – with one difference. In the loo, no one can hear you scream. Online, or in the post, as part of a national campaign, someone, somewhere may just hear your cry for help.

SEEKING COUNSELLING

There are many ways to access counselling. Your doctor may recommend it if your feelings are really starting to get on top of you or you're suffering stress overload. Some carers centres can put you in touch with a counsellor, or offer counselling sessions themselves. Or you can locate services privately in your area.

If there's nothing in the phone book, contact the British Association for Counselling who'll be able to give you the names of accredited professionals in your area. And don't be put off if you live in the back of beyond. Some agencies now offer counselling sessions over the phone.

Deciding to have a few counselling sessions may feel like a big step for a coper, but it's really no different from asking a doctor for help with a medical problem you can't resolve by yourself. The important thing to remember is to be absolutely clear with yourself and the counsellor why you are there. This is almost certainly not the time to be digging deep, looking back at all the things in your past which are now part of your DNA. What you need from these sessions is an emotional workout that will help you deal with your situation now.

Many counselling services are run by charities who are happy to work for a heavily subsidised rate with people on low incomes. Usually you'll be asked to agree with your counsellor what you can afford. The service may even be free of charge if you're referred by a doctor or by another professional. And don't forget the Samaritans, whose phone line operates 24 hours a day, seven days a week. Their trained volunteers are there to listen to anyone in distress or in need of emotional support.

ASK THE FAMILY, PHONE A FRIEND

There are any number of reasons why you may feel you're not getting support from other relatives or friends for you or the person you're caring for. The least charitable explanation is that they're just darn lazy and quite happy for you to carry the load, thank you very much. But, let's be honest, although we all know such sloths, the majority of people are basically decent; just busy and stressed and trying to juggle their commitments the same as you are.

And perhaps just a little worried – as they look at you – that if they raise their head above the parapet by offering to do something they'll be drawn in and end up carrying the lot – or at least far more than they bargained for.

The answer is to involve a lot of people in doing little things – which adds up to a decent amount of help for you. For instance, if your relatives always phone you for news of the person you're caring for, couldn't you agree to make just one call to one relative and then they can pass the news on to everyone else?

Take a look at some of the suggestions below for ways in which others might help, and add your own items or start your own list. By producing it you are making it safe for people to offer a hand, giving them the chance to choose to support you in a way that fits in with their lives.

You can also show the list, or suggest items from it, to those friends who offer to help. Remember, most people are genuine . . . and if the boot was on the other foot and you could see one of your friends going under, wouldn't you be first in the queue with a homemade casserole or a handkerchief?

HELP LIST

◆ Spare a few hours once a fortnight to sit with my loved one so I can get out.

◆ Take them for a drive from time to time.

◆ Come and read to them from a book or the newspaper on a regular basis.

◆ Bring cards or a board game to play with them.

◆ Bring a pet to visit.

◆ Do my shopping.

◆ Clean the car.

◆ Make an extra portion of dinner to put in the freezer for my loved one.

◆ Help with the gardening.

◆ Help with the housework.

◆ Take my children for an outing.

◆ Bring books and music from the library and then change them regularly.

SUPPORT FOR YOU: WHAT OTHER CARERS SAY

'The carers' group paid for me to do a creative writing course with the National Extension College and loaned a computer so I could write poetry and short stories. When you first go you think they're all going to be down and miserable but they're not at all. Most of the people I've met have a lot of energy and don't feel sorry for themselves at all.' **Maurice**

'We get ideas from each other. This chap has a mentally ill daughter who's lying in bed all the time and I said so was my son so I moved his bed into another room, away from the telly and computer. A week later he said that worked – she has to get up now.' **Jenny**

'My mum, nan and grandad, who I'd been caring for, died within five weeks of each other and I had a series of panic attacks. I was at A & E every week thinking I was having a heart attack. The doctor suggested a counsellor and to start with I bit her head off because she was trying to tell me I was suffering from stress! Of course before long I knew she was right: she's really helped me see what was wrong.' **Teresa**

14

Reviewing Where You Are

Bernadette cared for her father for more than a decade while her three sisters got on with having families, jobs and social lives. It wasn't that they loved their father less; simply that one by one they left home to get married until Bernadette was the only one still living with their father.

The unthinkable happened when her sisters, conscious that Bernadette was nearing breaking point, arranged cover for a fortnight so she could have her first proper holiday. A few days into a walking tour of France, Bernadette stayed in a remote country house run by a dynamic American. By the time the group was to move on to its next lodging, Bernadette and the landlord were in love. Back home, she told her sisters that after 10 years as their father's carer, she was going to get married and live in France and together they would need to make other care arrangements for their father.

The moral of this story is that no matter how tied you feel to the current care arrangements, there is always an alternative. It's just that we usually don't allow ourselves to see it until it rises up and smacks us in the face. If you suddenly announced you couldn't go on, someone, somewhere, most probably within the professional health and social services, would have to pick up the pieces.

Most of us don't encounter such dramatic life changes as Bernadette – but it is important to recognise that nothing in life stays the same and you need to keep reviewing your choices and asking yourself whether they are still working – for the person you care for, but especially for you.

HAS ANYTHING ALTERED?

When we're under pressure it usually feels easier to stick with what's familiar, to go on doing the same thing rather than try to summon the energy and space to alter anything. But there are some important reasons for looking at your role as a carer and all that it means. For instance:

◆ The decisions you made for your loved one's care may have been rushed by circumstances. In the light of experience and without that urgency, do they still look like the right decisions?

◆ Life moves on. Perhaps the person you're caring for needs more help or less help than they did. Are the arrangements you made still best for them and you?

◆ And what about all the other parts of your life: family, friends, dependants, work? Has anything changed there which you now need to take into account?

◆ Perhaps when you started caring you didn't know there were alternatives or that it might be possible to get more help. Are there changes that would benefit one or both of you?

REVIEWING YOUR CHOICES

The questions below are intended to guide your thoughts but they do cover some areas that you may find difficult, or may make you feel emotional. If so, try and get help working through the list, either from a trusted friend or from a professional such as a counsellor. You may also need to get help making changes which you realise you need to make once you've done your review. Turn back to the last chapter for some ideas about where to look.

QUESTIONS TO ASK YOURSELF

◆ What effect is being a carer having on you, your health, your social life, your plans for your own life?

◆ What effect is being a carer having on your job or career?

◆ What impact is caring having on your income – can you afford to continue?

◆ How is your caring affecting other members of your family and your relationships with them?

◆ How is being a carer affecting your relationship with the person you're caring for?

◆ Is their condition getting any worse?

◆ How much longer do you think you will need to be a carer?

◆ Is it likely that the demands on you will increase?

◆ If they do, do you think you can cope?

◆ Do you feel you are coping now?

◆ What alternatives are available to you?

Residential Care

Sometimes as carers we reach the point of deciding it's time to move the one we're caring for into a residential home. But even if you're certain the time has come to consider residential care for the person you care for – and few carers are sufficiently detached from their own situation to see it quite so clearly – your resolve is likely to be clouded by feelings of sadness, loss and guilt (especially if your loved one has told you they don't want to 'go into a home'). You may even feel that you have failed. Shouldn't you have been able to manage things in such a way that the person you've been caring for could continue to be cared for at home? Aren't you being selfish? Won't they be getting second-rate care if you're not there to deliver it?

Your feelings are understandable – and familiar to all those carers who've ventured down this route before you. You may find it helps to share your feelings with someone who has personal experience of what you're now going through. A carer support group may be able to put you in touch with others, or, when you start looking at residential homes, you can ask the home to put you in contact with the families of residents who are already there.

Remember, you have reached this point after looking at the impact of your caring role on everyone who is involved. What's in your best interests is almost certain to be in the best interests of others too. The other important thing to remember is that even if the person you care for goes into a nursing home, assisted accommodation, or any other residential care setting, you haven't stopped being a carer – any more than your children leaving home means you're no longer a parent. What it does mean is that you've got more time and energy for the best bits of a caring role: spending time with your loved one, talking, sharing an activity, sharing memories or sharing feelings, while someone else is dealing with the day-to-day.

No one is asking you to stop caring about the quality of care the person you've looked after now gets. You'll be a point of liaison for whatever residential setting you choose, and any such setting worth its salt will positively welcome your involvement and your vast experience of caring for your loved one.

CHOOSING RESIDENTIAL CARE

There are a whole range of things to consider when choosing any new 'home'. And it's unlikely that you'll be able to cover everything in a single visit. Indeed, visiting any of the places you're considering at different times of day, with different staff on duty and other routines underway, will give you a more accurate picture of the quality and consistency of care each is offering.

To frame your inspection and decision-making, these are just some of the things you might want to think about or ask:

- How does the person you're caring for feel about it?
- Do *you* like it? How would *you* feel about living there?
- Is it registered with a national or local association?
- What's the food like – can you both stay for a meal one day?
- Are visiting hours and numbers limited?
- Is it nicely decorated and is it clean?

◆ Does the home keep any pets or allow people to bring in their own?

◆ How practical will it be for you and other family and friends to visit (distance, public transport routes, etc.)?

◆ How will the place be paid for? Can you afford it?

◆ Can you get a clear breakdown of costs (some homes charge heavily for extras)?

◆ Is there a recent inspection report you can see?

◆ Can the home put you in touch with the families of other residents for references?

◆ If your loved one's condition gets worse do they have the facilities to keep them there? You don't want them to have to move again.

◆ What does the daily timetable look like? What activities and services are available?

◆ How many of the staff are permanent and how many agency (which may mean lots of different faces all the time)?

◆ Can your loved one bring in their own items to make the space more personal?

◆ Does the home have a waiting list? If so, how long (no point getting your hopes up)?

◆ Is there a contract you have to sign and what does this commit you to?

CONTINUING TO CARE

You may not be able to make it perfectly alright for your loved one if they hate the idea of leaving their own home or yours. But choosing a setting where they can take the things that matter to them and where they retain a degree of autonomy will give you the best chance of the new arrangements working.

Bear in mind that neither of you should rush to judgement. Finding the right setting and moving into it is a huge thing for you both and it may take months before life settles down enough for you to be able to judge whether the new arrangements are working. Hard as it may be, you need to hold your nerve until that point and be clear with your loved one that change is difficult for everyone and you both need time to get used to it.

In the meantime make a point of getting to know those who have taken on the caring role as you would if they were coming into your home. You are still a part of a caring partnership and playing an active role in it will make it easier for you to spot any problems, raise any issues, and act as your loved one's advocate.

Letting go may be very hard for you. But it is a mistake to spend too much time with the person you care for in the early days thinking you can withdraw a little once they've settled in. Having you there all the time will slow the process of them adapting to their new situation, and, believe me, you'll find it gets harder rather than easier to cut the time you spend there.

There are other ways of showing you care and are watching, apart from spending every minute of your spare time at their side. You can phone or drop them a note from time to time: everyone enjoys getting post. And now's also a good time to enlist help from others. It may be easier for other relatives to visit because they no longer have to feel so guilty that you're the one carrying the load.

16

Beyond Caring

One in every two of you reading this will be a carer for up to five years. Another 25 per cent of carers are involved in looking after someone for between five and 10 years, while the final 25 per cent are carers for over 10 years.

Whichever way you look at it, that's a big chunk out of anyone's life: long enough for different routines to have become ingrained, for your ideas and priorities to have changed. In short, for the world to look a very different place to the one you inhabited before you became a carer.

Many carers find the weeks, months and even years after their caring role ends as tough and emotional as what went before. They need help adjusting – and recognising there is something for them beyond caring.

AN END TO CARING

Your caring role may end for a number of reasons: the person you've been looking after may die; you may be a young carer who is leaving the nest to go to college, take up a job, or start your own family; you may be a parent carer who's had to make arrangements for your child to be more independent by moving them into a supported living environment. Whatever the reason, be prepared for some fallout, and allow yourself time coming to terms with what has happened.

You are facing more loss – which has been the theme of your life for a long time. However relieved you are to be free of some of the day-to-day practicalities, you are facing the loss of a close caring relationship and the loss of a role which, even if you hated it, you were at least familiar with.

For some the loss runs deeper still. After such an intense period pouring their energy into keeping someone else going, putting their own needs second, some people find they have lost sight of who they really are and how to go on with their own lives: their identity as a separate person.

WHEN THE ONE YOU ARE CARING FOR DIES

There are no rules about dying. The best any of us can hope for is a 'good death' and as a carer you will be doing your best to achieve that for the person you care for, whether you are nursing them through many years of slow decline, or a swift illness.

As part of that process, you may feel able to discuss with them their dying, their wishes for the way they are cared for up to their death and what they want to happen afterwards. Only you can judge that. In other cases, you may sense that this is not something you'll be able to discuss, or their condition may not allow you to. If so, it's important that you find someone with whom you can share your feelings, worries and practical concerns. Because your role brings you so close to the one you're caring for, you are, to a great extent, experiencing their dying with them. You need an outlet for all of the difficult emotions that will bring up for you.

If you don't have friends or a partner to share what you're feeling with, contact one of the excellent bereavement counselling charities: you'll find their details in the resources section at the back of this guide. Some carers centres run special programmes for 'former carers'.

Those carers who have been able to talk about dying with the one they're caring for often find great comfort and relief in it. At a practical level, knowing what last services you can do for someone you've cared for feels like completing the circle. At an emotional level, your honesty at this time may bring you still closer, cementing what has been – for good or ill – one of life's most significant relationships for you both.

You may want to talk about how they wish to spend their last weeks, people they want to see, even places they may want to visit. If they're suffering from a terminal illness, you may want to discuss pain control and whether they wish to be revived should something happen. They may want to share what they are feeling with you, their fears, or that they are ready to die. You could discuss funeral arrangements, where they would like to be buried or have their ashes scattered.

Equally, there may be times when neither of you wants to talk, simply to share the silence together. Don't be scared of silence. You have been so busy for so long that you may find it hard to sit quietly. But this really is a time when sharing peace is an important stage in the journey ending and beginning for you both.

WHAT TO DO WHEN SOMEONE DIES

Once upon a time most people died at home and we all grew up knowing what to do. These days we have less contact with death and its after-math. The checklist below will help you know what steps you must take, but don't be afraid to ask your doctor or a funeral director if you're worried or unclear.

Call the doctor

The doctor has to confirm the death and will write out a medical certificate saying what caused it. If your loved one dies in hospital then one of the hospital's medical staff will do this.

Contact a funeral director

If you have access to the will or to its executors, then look at this before you contact a funeral director to ensure you're aware of any special wishes. You should also consult any relatives who may want a say in the arrangements. Then find a funeral director – personal recommendation is the best way to choose. The funeral director will take much of the load from you if you wish, guiding you through your choices, contacting the crematorium, or other religious centre, for you, arranging flowers and placing a notice in the paper. It's best to go into the funeral home with an idea of what you can afford to spend: don't feel pressured into spending more than you want on expensive coffins and extras.

Register the death

You need to do this within five days of the death and at the registrar's office within whose district your loved one died. If in doubt, contact your local council or library for details. You'll need to take the medical certificate of death that the doctor wrote, plus the following documents if you have them: their birth and marriage certificates, medical card, pension or benefit books and details of any life insurance policies. The registrar will want to know your loved one's full name (including maiden name if appropriate), last address, date and place of birth, date and place of death, their occupation, details of any benefits they were receiving including pension, if they were married, the name and occupation of their husband or wife and any previous marriage partners, and the name and date of birth of any marriage partner surviving them. You'll be given a death certificate, a certificate for burial or cremation and a certificate of registration of death.

Arrange the funeral

The funeral can take place once you have given the certificate for burial or cremation to the funeral director. When it comes to the service itself, try to ensure it reflects a whole life rather than just the recent years of caring. Your loved one was not only a dependant, just as you are not only a carer.

Deal with the paperwork

You will need copies of the death certificate for when you contact any solicitors, banks and building societies and insurance companies to tie up loose ends. You should also contact the Benefits Agency to cancel pension or any other allowances. And if no one is going to be living in their house now, contact the services such as gas, electricity, water and phone companies, and the local council about Council Tax.

RIDING THE EMOTIONAL ROLLER COASTER

One of the effects of all this activity is to take your mind off both your loss and your future so don't be surprised if you don't feel the need to grieve straight away. Some carers feel guilty because they think they should be more upset. Others worry that because they feel fine, even relieved, they couldn't have loved the one they've just lost enough.

This is equally true if you've stopped being a carer for reasons other than death; for example, if the person you were caring for has moved into a new setting and is being cared for by others. There is a flurry of activity around making the new arrangements and winding up old ones, all of which postpones the moment when it is just you, and the silence, and the knowledge that your life is going to be different from now on.

It's important you tell yourself that whatever you're feeling at this stage is OK and very normal. You have been through a huge amount. Your body and mind need time and space to process this before you can begin to think about the future.

Loss and bereavement have their own patterns and timetables for each of us. It is normal to feel pain, sadness, anger, to experience denial – disbelief that anything has changed – and for your emotions to rise and fall as if you were on some kind of horrible roller coaster.

One of the first things you may experience is a sense of relief. Have you ever played that game where you stand in the doorway and push your arms out against the frame? When you stop, your arms fly up of their own accord, like wings. Ceasing to be a carer can feel like that. The pressure is off and the sense of light-headedness is intoxicating.

And yet after a few moments your limbs fall back to your side, as heavy as ever. On the emotional roller coaster there's a down for every up, every positive feeling has its opposite. You need to go with all those emotions, allowing them to run their course, and using the following to guide you.

TIPS

- Talk through the pain to those close to you as much as you need to. Expressing our feelings over and over again is our way of working through them.

- Be gentle with yourself. All the time you were a carer you were putting other people ahead of you. Now it really is time to take care of yourself.

- Don't be afraid of your emotions. They may be all over the place. You may be weeping one moment, angry another, and laughing the next as you recall something funny from the past. Whatever you feel is OK.

◆ Honour your memories. Hopefully there were some good times as well as bad times and both are now part of who you are. Even if you haven't got many good memories, remind yourself why you were a carer and honour what you were able to give in that role.

Be aware, however, that if the roller coaster seems endless and shows no sign of slowing down, or you realise that no matter how much you talk the pain never seems to get any less, you may need professional support. To grieve is normal; to be incapacitated by grief means you need help – which is not your fault, simply a reflection of how deeply being a carer has affected you.

FACING UP TO THE FUTURE

You may have given up a great deal to be a carer: your job or at least your chances of a career, your friendships, hobbies, interests, holidays. The list goes on and on. If so, the future may, for a while, look very scary indeed. So many minutes to fill, and you have very little idea of what to do with them. At first you think how much you'll enjoy taking yourself off for a walk in the park or a coffee with friends but there's less pleasure in it than you'd expected. You're so used to being busy you can't adjust to having nowhere you need to be, nothing that desperately needs to be done.

Some carers experience a loss even deeper than loss of their carer role. Having lived on the borders of someone else's life rather than at the centre of their own, they have lost the direction they once had and are left wondering what to do with their lives. For other carers, the huge 'what next?' question mark hovering over their heads is simply pragmatism. If 10 or 20 years have gone by since you started caring you may well no longer want the same things you did long ago. The world of work may have moved on and left you behind. Being a carer may have changed what you want out of life and you simply haven't had time to think about putting any other dreams or ambitions in place of old ones that are now redundant.

Do think about getting help at this crucial time. All of a sudden, the social workers, care assistants, home helps and health professionals who offered you at least a little support have vanished from your life. But there are others able to step into the gap and ensure that you're cared for. Many carers centres run special groups for 'former carers' precisely because they know how critical it is that carers are helped to adjust. Counselling agencies or bereavement counselling may also be useful at this time.

You do have a future and you're owed help deciding what it will look like. Keep this checklist close by and consult it often.

CARE PLAN FOR CARERS

- ◆ **Do** get support from friends, counsellors and carer support groups.

- ◆ **Do** consult your doctor if you think you need medical help, for instance if you feel exhausted all the time or feel depressed.

- ◆ **Do** get lots of rest. However well you've managed, your batteries are in need of comprehensive recharging.

- ◆ **Do** make plans for difficult days if the person you cared for has died. Birthdays and anniversaries can be specially difficult and you need to spend them with people who will understand your mixed emotions and be willing to listen.

- ◆ **Do** get a health check: your health may have suffered or been neglected. It's time to focus on you.

◆ **Don't** make any decisions about the future quickly. You need to deal with things in your own time.

◆ **Don't** let anyone tell you you must be glad it's all over. Your feelings are far more complex than that.

◆ **Don't** worry if you suffer 'relapses'. Few of us live our emotional lives in a straight line.

◆ **Don't** reproach yourself that you could have done more. You did the best you could at the time.

PAST CARING: WHAT OTHER CARERS SAY

'Did I get anything out of it? Yes, I think it made me appreciate the little things – trees, the sky, grass, colours – which a lot of people don't see because they have to go out to work to pay the mortgage and they have to work so hard. When I did get time away it was like seeing life through a different pair of eyes.' **Rose**

'I was her rock, but I never realised how much she was my rock too. So when she died I was totally, totally lost. I knew I could go anywhere and do anything . . . but I didn't and I don't.' **Janet**

'I dread being cared for. I had to deal with all the womanly things for Kim and I dread that kind of intrusion. I've said to my kids if that ever happens to me put a pillow over my head but don't get caught. And in a way I'm serious.' **Tony**

'For the remaining months of his life we were totally at peace and comfortable together. No more self-consciousness. No unfinished business . . . In a way this was my father's final gift to me: the chance to see him as something more than my father; the chance to see the common identity of spirit we both shared.' **Ram Dass** in *How can I help?*

Resources

Many of the organisations that appear below have separate offices in England, Scotland, Wales and Northern Ireland. Many also have an extensive network of regional or local branches. To simplify this section for readers, I have, in most cases, given contact details for the organisation's headquarters, from whom you'll get up-to-date information on services in your part of the UK.

NATIONAL CARER ORGANISATIONS

The Princess Royal Trust for Carers
Tel: 020 7480 7788
www.carers.org

London Office:
142 Minories
London EC3N 1LB
info@carers.org

Glasgow Office:
Charles Oakley House
125 West Regent Street
Glasgow G2 2SD
Tel: 0141 221 5066
infoscotland@carers.org

Wales Office:
104 Mansel Street
Swansea SA1 5UE
Tel: 01792 472908

*The Princess Royal Trust for Carers is the largest provider of com-
prehensive carers support services in the UK. Through its network of
130 independently managed carers centres, and its websites,* carers.org
and youngcarers.net, *it provides quality information, advice and support
services to 290,000 carers, including 15,000 young carers.*

Carers UK
CarersLine: 0808 808 7777
www.carersuk.org

20-25 Glasshouse Yard
London EC1A 4JT
Tel: 020 7490 8818

Carers Scotland
91 Mitchell Street
Glasgow G1 3LN
Tel: 0141 221 9141
info@carerscotland.org

Carers Wales
River House
Ynsbridge Court
Gwaelod-y-Garth
Cardiff CF15 9SS
info@carerswales.org

Carers Northern Ireland
58 Howard Street
Belfast BT1 6PJ
Tel: 028 9043 9843
info@carersni.org

Carers UK is an organisation of carers fighting on behalf of carers for a better deal. Alongside its campaigns it offers information, advice and forums for carers, plus high quality courses for health and social care professionals, advice workers, employers and anyone who works with carers.

Crossroads Caring for Carers
Tel: 0845 450 0350
www.crossroads.org.uk

Crossroads Association
10 Regent Place
Rugby
Warwickshire CV21 2PN

Crossroads runs schemes in most parts of England and Wales to provide trained carer support workers to take over from carers so they can have a break.

YOUNG CARERS
Young Carers
www.youngcarers.net

Website for young carers, run by the Princess Royal Trust for Carers (see p. 147–8 for contacts).

RESOURCES AND SUPPORT FOR CARERS

BackCare
Helpline: 0845 130 2704
www.backpain.org

16 Elmtree Road
Teddington
Middlesex TW11 8ST

Help with the prevention and management of back pain.

British Red Cross
Tel: 0870 170 7000
www.redcross.org.uk

UK Office
44 Moorfields
London EC2Y 9AL

Care in the home, day care centres, assistance with transport, first aid training, loan of medical aids and equipment.

Counsel and Care
Helpline: 0845 300 7585
www.counselandcare.org.uk

Tyman House
16 Bonny Street
London NW1 9PG

Advice for people over 60, their families and carers, on all aspects of community care, including: services for older people, residential and nursing homes, hospital discharge, claiming benefits, carers issues and living at home.

Department of Health
Main customer service line: 020 7210 4850
www.dh.gov.uk

Department of Health
Richmond House
79 Whitehall
London SW1A 2NS

Fund of information on health and social care issues, publications and advice, plus links to other useful helplines.

DirectGov
www.direct.gov.uk

The UK goverment's website-based information service aiming to make it easier for people to access a huge range of information and services in one location – including comprehensive sections on benefits, pensions, health, parenting and employment. Of special interest to carers are the quick links to www.direct.gov.uk/CaringForSomeone and www.direct.gov.uk/ DisabledPeople.

NHS Direct
Tel: 0845 4647
www.nhsdirect.nhs.uk

24-hour nurse advice and health information service, run by the NHS as a first stop for the diagnosis and treatment of common conditions.

Royal British Legion
Legionline: 0845 7725 725
www.britishlegion.org.uk

48 Pall Mall
London SW1Y 5JY

Financial, social and emotional support to servicemen and women and their dependants, including grant-making, counselling, job retraining, home and hospital visits and full nursing care.

SSAFA (Soldiers, Sailors, Airmen and Families Association)
Tel: 020 7403 8783
www.ssafa.org.uk

19 Queen Elizabeth St
London SE1 2LP
info@ssafa.org.uk

Financial, practical and emotional support for former and serving servicemen and women and their families. SSAFA's services are provided through a network of 7,000 volunteers.

United Kingdom Home Care Association
Tel: 020 8288 1551
www.ukhca.co.uk

Group House
2nd Floor
52 Sutton Court Road
Sutton
Surrey SM1 4SL
helpline@ukhca.co.uk

Advice on choosing care and searchable database of organisations providing care – including nursing and live-in care – to people in their own homes.

UK Self Help
www.ukselfhelp.info

Internet database with details of over 800 UK self-help groups and support organisations providing advice, information and empathy for more than 2,000 needs, conditions and diseases.

MONEY

Benefits Enquiry Line
Helpline: 0800 882200
Textphone: 0800 24 33 55

Confidential advice and information for people with disabilities and their carers about social security benefits and how to claim them.

Citizens Advice Bureau
Visit the website or see phone book for details of nearest local centre
www.citizensadvice.org.uk
Online information: www.adviceguide.org.uk

Free, independent source of advice on legal, benefits and other problems through UK-wide network of branches.

Community Legal Services Direct
Tel: 0845 345 4345
www.clsdirect.org.uk

Information and advice on the legal and financial aspects of looking after someone else's affairs.

Department for Constitutional Affairs
Tel: 020 7210 8500
www.dca.gov.uk

Selborne House
54 Victoria Street
London SW1E 6QW
United Kingdom

Advice and publications on Power of Attorney, the Court of Protection and other aspects of looking after someone else's affairs.

Family Fund
Tel: 0845 130 45 42
www.familyfund.org.uk

Family Fund
4 Alpha Court
Monks Cross Drive
Huntington
York YO32 9WN
info@familyfund.org.uk

The Family Fund helps families in the UK caring for a severely disabled child living at home. It provides grants related to the needs of that child, provided they are under 15 and meet certain criteria.

Independent Review Service
Tel: 0800 096 1296
www.irs-review.org.uk

4th Floor
City Podium
5 Hill Street
Birmingham B5 4UB

*Deals independently with carers' appeals if applications to the Social
Fund – administered by JobCentre Plus – are turned down.*

The Pension Service
National helpline: 0845 6060 265
www.thepensionservice.gov.uk (England, Scotland and Wales)
www.dsdni.gov.uk (for Northern Ireland)

Pensions Direct
Tyneview Park
Whitley Road
Benton
Newcastle-upon-Tyne NE98 1BA

*Part of the Department of Work and Pensions, provides information and
advice on all aspects of saving for and claiming a pension.*

EMPLOYMENT, EDUCATION AND TRAINING

ACE
Advice line: 0808 800 5793
www.ace-ed.org.uk

*Independent advice centre offering information about state education
in England and Wales to parents of 5-16 year olds including those with
special educational needs.*

Employers for Carers

www.carersuk.org/Employersforcarers

European Social Fund-supported project bringing together Carers UK and major employers to encourage and offer advice to other employers on introducing more carer-friendly working practices.

Jobcentre Plus

See phone book for contact details of your nearest centre
Jobseeker Direct line: 0845 6060 234
www.jobcentreplus.gov.uk

Part of the Department of Work and Pensions, provides help and advice on jobs and training for people who can work, and financial help for those who can't.

Learn Direct

Tel: 0800 100900
www.learndirect.co.uk

Information on over 1,500 local learndirect centres, plus impartial advice on over 900,000 courses, including their own specially created online courses you can study at a time and pace to suit you.

Learning and Skills Council

Helpline: 0870 900 6800
www.lsc.gov.uk

Advice on local LSCs who can provide information on local post-education training opportunities, other than university.

Learning for Living
www.learningforliving.co.uk

Online course developed by carers for carers, offering both information and support, and a qualification.

Listening Books
Tel: 020 7407 9417
www.listening-books.org.uk

12 Lant Street
London SE1 1QH

Postal audio library book service for people who have difficulty reading in the usual way.

National Extension College
01223 400 200
www.nec.ac.uk

Michael Young Centre
Purbeck Road
Cambridge CB2 2HN

Wide range of courses available for home study, including GSCE, A level, professional and personal interest programmes.

Open University
Tel: 0845 300 60 90
www.open.ac.uk

PO Box 724

Milton Keynes MK7 6ZS

Biggest selection of courses for home study, from short courses in creative writing and family history through to degree and postgraduate level study. Financial support often available for the low and unwaged.

U3A (University of the Third Age)
Tel: 020 8466 6139
www.u3a.org.uk

Provides lifelong learning opportunities for those no longer in gainful employment, through a network of local groups and online courses. Phone or see website for nearest group.

Working Families
Helpline: 0800 013 0313
www.workingfamilies.org.uk
edads@workingfamilies.org.uk

1-3 Berry Street
London EC1V 0AA

Information, advice, factsheets and ongoing support for parents and carers on: parental leave, tax credits and benefits, time off for emergencies, childcare and flexible working. Network and newsletter for families with disabled children.

HOLIDAYS AND RESPITE CARE

Hospice Information
Helpline: 0870 903 3903
www.hospiceinformation.info

Help the Hospices
Hospice House
34-44 Britannia Street
London WC1X 9JG

Information service for the public and professionals on hospices and palliative care (caring for dying people).

Leonard Cheshire
Tel: 020 7802 8200
www.leonard-cheshire.org

30 Millbank
London SW1P 4QD

Supporting disabled people through a wide range of services, including care at home services, respite and day services for disabled people and their carers, and rehabilitation.

Tourism for All UK
Tel: 0845 124 9971
www.tourismforall.org.uk
info@tourismforall.org.uk

c/o Vitalise
Shap Road Industrial Estate
Kendal
Cumbria LA9 6NZ

Tourism for All (formerly Holiday Care) is the UK's central source of holiday and travel information for disabled people and their carers, including: accessible accommodation, visitor attractions and transport, activity holidays, holidays with children, respite care and sources of funding.

Vitalise (formerly Winged Fellowship Trust)
Tel: 0845 345 1972
Bookings line: 0845 345 1970
www.vitalise.org.uk
bookings@vitalise.org.uk

12 City Forum
250 City Road
London EC1V 8AF

Breaks for disabled people and carers at five fully accessible UK centres.

COUNSELLING

British Association for Counselling and Psychotherapy
Tel: 0870 443 5252
www.bacp.co.uk

BACP House
15 St John's Business Park
Lutterworth
Leicestershire LE17 4HB

Directory of therapists operating in your area.

Relate
See phone book for your nearest local centre.
Tel: 0845 4561310
www.relate.org.uk

Federation of local centres supporting couple and family relationships through counselling, sex therapy and relationship education.

Samaritans
Tel: 08457 90 90 90
www.samaritans.org

write to: Chris
PO Box 9090
Stirling FK8 2SA
jo@samaritans.org

24-hour helpline for anyone in distress, despair or in need of emotional support.

BEREAVEMENT

The Compassionate Friends
Helpline: 0845 123 2304
www.tcf.org.uk

53 North St
Bristol BS3 1EN
helpline@tcf.org.uk

Offers support, understanding and advice to parents and families after the death of a child; and to those helping the family.

Cruse Bereavement Care
Helpline: 0870 167 1677
Young Person's Helpline: 0808 808 1677
www.crusebereavementcare.org.uk

Cruse House
126 Sheen Road
Richmond
Surrey TW9 1UR

Counselling and support for bereaved people, plus information, advice, education and training services.

The Way Foundation
Tel: 0870 011 3450
www.wayfoundation.org.uk

PO Box 6767
Brackley NN13 6YW

Self-help social and support network for men and women widowed up to the age of 50 and their children.

Winstons Wish
Helpline: 0845 203 04 05
www.winstonswish.org.uk

Clara Burgess Centre
Bayshill Rd
Cheltenham
Glos GL50 3AW

Practical support and guidance for children and young people who have been bereaved of a close family member.

DISABILITY AIDS AND MOBILITY

DIAL UK
Tel: 01302 310123
www.dialuk.info

St Catherine's
Tickhill Road
Doncaster
South Yorkshire
DN4 8QN

National organisation for network of 140 local disability information and advice services, run by and for disabled people.

Disabled Living Foundation
Helpline: 0845 139 9177
www.dlf.org.uk

380-384 Harrow Road
London W9 2HU

National charity running free, impartial advice about all types of disability aids, equipment and mobility products.

Motability
Tel: 0845 456 4566
www.motability.co.uk

Warwick House
Roydon Road
Harlow
Essex CM19 5PX

+Provides affordable, convenient, trouble-free motoring to over 440,000 disabled customers and their families. Powered wheelchairs and scooters can be financed using the Motability scheme.

The Mobility Market
Tel: 0161 788 8676
www.themobilitymarket.co.uk

Dolphin House
36 Liverpool Road
Eccles
Manchester M30 0WA

Established for the public to sell their unwanted, pre-owned mobility aids and disability equipment to others via an easy-to-use, secure and value-for-money service.

CHILDREN, YOUNG PEOPLE AND PARENTING

Childline
Helpline: 0800 1111
www.childline.org.uk

Free helpline for children and young people who need to talk to counsellors about any problem.

Contact A Family
Helpline: 0808 808 3555
www.cafamily.org.uk

209-211 City Road
London EC1V 1JN

Support and advice to parents whatever the medical condition of their child; the charity has information on over 1,000 rare syndromes and disorders and can often put families in touch with each other.

Gingerbread

Advice line: 0800 018 4318

www.gingerbread.org.uk

Gingerbread

307 Borough High Street

London SE1 1JH

Organistion for lone parent families offering friendship, support and advice.

Hyperactive Children's Support Group

Tel: 01243 539966

www.hacsg.org.uk

71 Whyke Lane

Chichester

West Sussex PO19 7PD

Information and support for the families of ADHD/hyperactive children.

SENIORS

Age Concern

Helpline: 0800 00 99 66

www.ageconcern.org.uk

Age Concern England
Astral House
1268 London Road
London SW16 4ER

Northern Ireland
Tel: 02890 24 5729
www.ageconcernni.org

Scotland
Tel: 0845 833 0200
www.ageconcernscotland.org.uk

Wales
Tel: 0800 00 9966
www.accymru.org.uk

*Day care, information and advice services for all people aged over 50,
operated through network of local centres.*

Help the Aged
Tel: 020 7278 1114
www.helptheaged.org.uk

207-221 Pentonville Road
London N1 9UZ

Northern Ireland
Tel: 02890 230 666

Scotland
Tel: 0131 551 6331

Wales

Tel: 02920 346 550

Support for older people, including advice on finances, housing, home safety and welfare rights.

MENTAL HEALTH

Mind

Infoline: 0845 766 0163

www.mind.org.uk

15-19 Broadway

London E15 4BQ

contact@mind.org.uk

Confidential help on a range of mental health issues and community services run through 200 local and regional centres.

Rethink (formerly National Schizophrenia Fellowship)

Tel: 0845 456 0455

www.rethink.org

5th Floor

Royal London House

22-25 Finsbury Square

London EC2A 1DX

Information and community services including employment projects, day services, supported housing, residential care and respite centres.

Sane
Helpline: 0845 767 8000
www.sane.org.uk

1st Floor
Cityside House
40 Adler Street
London E1 1EE

Support and information on all aspects of mental illness, including depression, manic depression, anxiety and schizophrenia.

INFORMATION AND SUPPORT GROUPS FOR SPECIFIC MEDICAL AND DISABILITY CONDITIONS

National Attention Deficit Disorder Information and Support Service (AD/HD) ADDISS
Tel: 020 8952 2800
www.addiss.co.uk

PO Box 340
Edgeware
Middlesex HA8 9HL

Information, resources and a helpline for parents, sufferers and health professionals on attention deficit hyperactivity disorder.

The Alzheimer's Society
Helpline: 0845 300 0336
www.alzheimers.org.uk

Gordon House
10 Greencoat Place
London SW1P 1PH

Information, advice, support and referrals to anyone with concerns about Alzheimer's disease or any other form of dementia, and to their families and carers.

Arthritis Care
Free helpline: 0808 800 4050
www.arthritiscare.org.uk

18 Stephenson Way
London NW1 2HD

Arthritis Care offers support and self-management training to help people of all ages with arthritis to lead full, independent lives. See the website for free, downloadable resources, information and for discussion forums.

National Autistic Society
Helpline: 0845 070 4004
www.autism.org.uk

393 City Road
London EC1V 1NG

Championing the rights of all people with autism and Asperger syndrome and ensuring they and their families receive quality services. The Society offers a range of services across the UK including schools, adult services, social groups, befrienders and advocacy.

(BLIND) Royal National Institute of the Blind
Helpline: 0845 766 9999
www.rnib.org.uk

105 Judd Street
London WC1H 9NE

Specialist advice and support services on all sight problems, plus aids, benefits, registering and links to local support groups and services.

Cancer Backup
Helpline: 0808 800 1234
www.cancerbackup.org.uk

3 Bath Place
Rivington Street
London EC2A 3JR

Information, practical advice and support for cancer patients and their families.

Colostomy Association
Helpline: 0800 587 6744
www.colostomyassociation.org.uk

15 Station Road
Reading
Berks RG1 1LG
cass@colostomyassociation.org.uk

Support, reassurance and practical information to ostomates and anyone about to have a colostomy.

The Continence Foundation
Helpline: 0845 345 0165
www.continence-foundation.org.uk

The Helpline Nurse
The Continence Foundation
307 Hatton Square
16 Baldwin Gardens
London EC1N 7RJ
(enclosing large SAE)

Information, advice and expertise on all aspects of continence.

Cystic Fibrosis Trust
Helpline: 0845 859 1000
www.cftrust.org.uk

11 London Road
Bromley
Kent BR1 1BY

Information, advice and support.

Diabetes UK
Careline: 0845 120 2960
www.diabetes.org.uk

Macleod House
10 Parkway
London NW1 7AA

Information and support on any aspect of managing diabetes: medication, diet, exercise, employment, driving, etc.

(DEAF) Royal National Institute of the Deaf
(for deaf and hard of hearing people)
Information line: 0808 808 0123
www.rnid.org.uk

19-23 Featherstone Street
London EC1Y 8SL

*Confidential and impartial information on tinnitus, employment, equip-
ment, legislation and benefits as well as issues relating to deafness and
hearing loss.*

Down's Syndrome Association
Helpline: 0845 230 0372
www.downs-syndrome.org.uk

Langdon Down Centre
2a Langdon Park
Teddington TW11 9PS

*Information and support for people with Down's syndrome, their families
and carers, plus referrals to local support groups.*

British Heart Foundation
Information line: 08450 70 80 70
www.bhf.org.uk

14 Fitzhardinge Street
London W1H 6DH

Information and advice on all aspects of heart health and disease.

Headway – the brain injury association
Helpline: 0808 800 2244
www.headway.org.uk

4 King Edward Court
King Edward Street
Nottingham NG1 1EW

Information, support and services to people with a brain injury, their family and carers.

(HIV) Terence Higgins Trust
Helpline: 0845 1221 200
www.tht.org.uk

214-230 Grays Inn Road
London WC1X 8DP

The Terence Higgins Trust is the UK's leading HIV and sexual health charity, providing a wide range of services across England, Wales and Scotland. The charity also campaigns for greater political and public understanding of the impact of HIV.

British Liver Trust
Tel: 0870 770 8028
www.britishlivertrust.org.uk

Portman House
44 High Street
Ringwood BH24 1AG

Information, support and advice to people concerned about or living with liver disease.

Macmillan Cancer Relief
Helpline: 0808 808 2020
www.macmillan.org.uk

89 Albert Embankment
London SE1 7UQ

Information, emotional support and local services on all aspects of cancer care and treatment for those with cancer and their families.

Marie Curie Cancer Care
Tel: 020 7599 7777
www.mariecurie.org.uk

89 Albert Embankment
London SE1 7TP

Best-known for its Marie Curie nurses, who provide care in the community for terminally ill cancer patients, plus practical and emotional support for them and their carers. Marie Curie also runs hospices and funds research.

(ME) Action for ME (Myalgic Encephalomyelitis/Encephalopathy)
Support line: 0845 123 2314
Welfare rights helpline: 01749 330136
www.afme.org.uk

Third Floor
Canningford House
38 Victoria Street
Bristol BS1 6BY

Factfiles, information, support and campaigning.

Mencap
Tel: 020 7454 0454
www.mencap.org.uk

123 Golden Lane
London EC1Y 0RT
information@mencap.org.uk

The UK's leading learning disability charity, working with people with a learning disability, their families and carers. Mencap fights to change laws and services to ensure people with a learning disability get an equal chance. It directly supports thousands of people to live their lives the way they want.

Motor Neurone Disease Association
Helpline: 08457 626262
www.mndassociation.org

PO Box 246
Northampton NN1 2PR

Information, support and advice for people with MND and their carers; some grants may be available.

Multiple Sclerosis Society
Helpline: 0808 800 8000
www.mssociety.org.uk

372 Edgware Road
London NW2 6ND

Runs respite care centres, provides financial assistance, and provides information and publications on MS, including support services for carers.

Parkinson's Disease Society
Free helpline: 0808 800 0303
www.parkinsons.org.uk

215 Vauxhall Bridge Road
London SW1V 1EJ

*The UK's leading authority on Parkinson's. Provides information and a
local support network for people with Parkinson's, their families, friends
and carers.*

Scope
Helpline: 0808 800 3333
www.scope.org.uk

Scope Response
PO Box 833
Milton Keynes MK12 5NY
(enclose SAE)

*Information, advice, and the chance to talk, for those living with cerebral
palsy and their families and carers.*

Sense
Tel: 020 7561 3384
www.sense.org.uk

11-13 Clifton Terrace
Finsbury Park
London N4 3SR

*Information, services and local support groups related to deaf-blindness
and associated disabilities, for all ages.*

SIA (Spinal Injuries Association)
Helpline: 0800 980 0501
www.spinal.co.uk

SIA House
2 Trueman Road
Oldbrook
Milton Keynes MK6 2HH

Sharing information and experience to help people lead a full life after injury.

Acknowledgements

I am immensely grateful to Jackie Ruane who cast a kind and expert eye on the manuscript, made many useful comments and suggestions, and kept me focused at several important stages along the way. My thanks too, to Harvey Brown and Katy Brown of the Milton Keynes Carers Project who were generous in sharing with me their experience of working with carers, put me in touch with many carers, and somehow also found time to read and comment on the manuscript.

For this second edition, Peter Tihanyi on behalf of The Princess Royal Trust for Carers kindly agreed to read and comment on the manuscript, alert me to changes, gaps, and sections which needed some clarification. I am very grateful to him and his colleagues at The Trust who continue to work on behalf of carers everywhere. In addition, the online resources of both The Princess Royal Trust for Carers and Carers UK, were once again invaluable, and I urge readers to use them, if only to reassure themselves that they are not alone.

I also owe thanks to Dawn Steel of The Open University and Annette Eden of Milton Keynes Welfare Rights, who looked at the sections on work and benefits, and delivered their comments and suggestions so expertly to meet a tight deadline. And to Judith Cameron, whose own experiences of being a carer in *The Guardian* helped make many of the issues I've written about in this book more real to other carers, and to the professionals reading the newspaper. I was delighted when she agreed to write a Foreword to this edition.

Many carers agreed to talk to me and I am grateful for their interest, but especially their honesty in sharing often very difficult experiences and emotions. Those who were happy to be credited by name in this guide are as follows: Tony Baxter, Ros Buckle, Linda Camborne-Paynter, Janet Cooper, Teresa Davidson, Jenny Doran, Martha Henderson, Carol Kenneally, Hazel Matthews, Mary McCabe, Devinder Panesar, Joyce Statham and Mary Wootton.

Finally, there were a number of books I found very useful in thinking about how to tackle this guide, what to put in and what to leave out. They are listed below.

Past Caring, Audrey Jenkinson (Promenade Publishing, 2003)
The Story of My Father, Sue Miller (Bloomsbury, 2004)
Which? Guide to Caring for Parents in Later Life (Which? 1992)
A Caregiver's Survival Guide, Kay Marshall Strom (InterVarsity Press, Illinois, 2000)
The Selfish Pig's Guide to Caring, Hugh Marriott (Polperro Heritage Press, 2003)
The 36-Hour Day (*caring for persons with Alzheimer disease and related dementing illness and memory loss in later life*), Nancy L. Mace, MA and Peter V. Rabins, MD, MPH (Warner Books, 1981)
C, John Diamond (Vermilion, 1998)
The Caregiver's Essential Handbook (*More than 1,200 Tips to help you care for Seniors*), Sandra Choron, MS and Sasha Carr (Contemporary Books, 2003)
Make the Most of Being a Carer, Ann Whitfield (Need2Know, 1996)
Hello and How are You? (Macmillan Cancer Relief, 2004)
Carer's Handbook (*Authorised manual of the Voluntary Aid Societies*) (Dorling Kindersley, 1997)

Index